ATLAS OF GALLIUM-67 SCINTIGRAPHY

A New Method of
Radionuclide Medical Diagnosis

ATLAS OF GALLIUM-67 SCINTIGRAPHY

A New Method of Radionuclide Medical Diagnosis

**Gerald S. Johnston
and A. Eric Jones**

*Department of Nuclear Medicine
Clinical Center
Department of Health, Education, and Welfare
National Institutes of Health
Bethesda, Maryland*

PLENUM PRESS • NEW YORK-LONDON

Library of Congress Cataloging in Publication Data

Johnston, Gerald S   1930-
    Atlas of gallium-67 scintigraphy.

    Bibliography: p.
    1. Radioisotope scanning—Atlases. 2. Gallium—Isotopes. 1. Jones, Alfred Eric,
1935-   joint author. II. Title [DNLM: 1. Gallium—Diagnostic use—Atlases. 2.
Neoplasms—Radiography—Atlases. 3. Radioisotope scanning—Atlases. WN17 J72a
1973]
RC78.7.R4J63   616.07'575   73-18375
ISBN-13: 978-1-4613-4498-8   e-ISBN-13: 978-1-4613-4496-4
DOI: 10.1007/978-1-4613-4496-4

Plenum Press is a Division of Plenum Publishing Corporation
227 West 17th Street, New York, N.Y. 10011

United Kingdom edition published by Plenum Press, London
A Division of Plenum Publishing Company, Ltd.
Davis House (4th Floor), 8 Scrubs Lane, Harlesden, London, NW10 6SE, England

CONTRIBUTORS

National Institutes of Health, Bethesda, Maryland

James C. Arseneau, M. D.
Medicine Branch, National Cancer Institute

Robert S. Frankel, M. D.
Department of Nuclear Medicine, Clinical Center

Louis G. Gelrud, M. D.
Section on Diseases of the Liver, Metabolic Diseases Branch,
National Institute of Arthritis, Metabolism and Digestive Diseases

Gerald S. Johnston, M. D.
Department of Nuclear Medicine, Clinical Center

Alfred E. Jones, M. D.
Department of Nuclear Medicine, Clinical Center

Robert J. Kramer, M. D.
Department of Nuclear Medicine, Clinical Center

Michael S. Milder, M. D.
Department of Nuclear Medicine, Clinical Center

Steven D. Richman, M. D.
Department of Nuclear Medicine, Clinical Center

PREFACE

In 1970, under the sponsorship of Oak Ridge Associated Universities (ORAU), a group of clinical investigators formed the Cooperative Group to Study Localization of Radiopharmaceuticals. The first radiopharmaceutical selected for study was 67-Gallium (67-Ga) administered as the citrate. The object of the study was to determine the usefulness of 67-Ga in the diagnosis and treatment of patients with various malignancies. Funding for the project was granted by the U. S. Atomic Energy Commission and the National Cancer Institute, National Institutes of Health (NIH). The Nuclear Medicine Department of the Clinical Center, NIH, agreed to assist ORAU with aspects of this study, particularly with 67-Ga scintigraphy of patients with lymphoma and Hodgkin's disease. Preliminary reports from the ORAU study are in press.

Since April 1971, 67-Ga scintigraphy has gained increasing use in the study of cancer patients at the Clinical Center, NIH, where well over 1000 such patients have been examined by this method. This monograph was written to present selected examples from this group of a variety of malignancies seen in this 28-month period. No attempt has been made to correlate this overall experience statistically. Rather, this presentation is to help familiarize the practitioner of Nuclear Medicine with the wide range of usefulness for 67-Ga scintigraphy while making him aware of the variation in scan appearance and watchful of the many pitfalls of 67-Ga scan interpretation.

Permission to use these patient studies and x-rays was generously granted by Dr. Paul P. Carbone, Associate Director, Medical Oncology, Division of Cancer Treatment, National Cancer Institute; Dr. John L. Doppman, Chief, Department of Radiology, Clinical Center; Dr. Alfred S. Ketcham, Clinical Director and Chief, Surgery Branch, National Cancer Institute; Dr. Ralph E. Johnson, Chief, Radiation Branch, National Cancer Institute; and Dr. John M. Van Buren, Chief, Surgical Neurology Branch, National Institute of Neurological Diseases and Stroke.

All scintigraphs were obtained with the expert technical help of Camille L. Boyce, Jeanne K. Honicker, Bonnie A. Mefferd, Eleanor J. Myers and Sybil J. Swann. The manuscript was typed by Luella Bentz, Paula McPherson, and Cathy S. Yarrison.

CONTENTS

CHAPTER 1

History and Method of Scan

Gerald S. Johnston, M. D.

Department of Nuclear Medicine, Clinical Center

National Institutes of Health, Bethesda, Maryland

In the late 1940's, radionuclides from the Oak Ridge reactor were made available for medical use. Up to that time, most nuclear medical experience had been with the application of phosphorus-32 (32-P) to hematologic diseases and iodine-131 (131-I) to thyroid problems. Both of these radionuclides were found to have valuable therapeutic applications in addition to their diagnostic uses.

Therapeutic "successes" with 32-P and 131-I helped encourage the hope that radionuclides would have important uses in cancer treatment. Among the radioactive agents studied to determine therapeutic usefulness were radioisotopes of gallium. These were examined for efficacy in the treatment of malignancies involving bone (1-5), and for usefulness in diagnosing bone involvement with tumor (3,4), and the presence of soft tumor (3). Toxic in high dosage, gallium-72 (72-Ga) did concentrate in bone tumors.

When 72-Ga was shown to be ineffective in the treatment of bone tumors, gallium-67 (67-Ga) was produced in a carrier-free state with the thought of increasing the amount of radioactivity that bone would concentrate by eliminating the carrier gallium which had produced toxic symptoms with 72-Ga (6). Surprisingly, the cyclotron produced, carrier-free 67-Ga had a different distribution in experimental animals than the high carrier reactor produced 67-Ga. 67-Ga did not accumulate in bones to any great extent, and so the therapeutic concentrations of this radionuclide could not be achieved in bony lesions. The addition of cold gallium to the 67-Ga in amounts equivalent to that found with 72-Ga resulted in similar 72-Ga and 67-Ga characteristics, but the cold gallium returned the problem of toxicity. Two patterns of gallium

concentration were thus established, that with carrier-free 67-Ga
and that with cold gallium carrier in amounts above 0.25 mg/kg
body weight mixed with 67-Ga. This latter gives the same pattern
observed with carrier containing 72-Ga (6). Similar observations
were made for 68-Ga (7). However, the studies previously done with
high carrier 72-Ga were not repeated with carrier-free 67-Ga or
68-Ga at the time these latter two isotopes became available.

Increased experience with radionuclides in medicine soon
indicated that the many hoped-for therapeutic applications were
not at hand. Instead, the possibilities of diagnostic uses for
radionuclides were emerging one after another. The hope then arose
that a tumor-localizing agent would be found to help with the
diagnosis and staging of cancer. Gallium isotopes faded into the
background temporarily as having no readily apparent use in nuclear
medicine.

With technological advances in the field, bone imaging emerged
as a valuable diagnostic method in the 1960's. Strontium-85 was
found to localize readily in areas of osteoblastic activity present
in primary and metastatic bone lesions (8). However, the long
half-life and energetic photon of 85-Sr were not satisfactory, and
the search continued for a better bone imaging agent. Fluorine-18
met the need for a shorter lived bone seeking nuclide (9), but it
was difficult to deliver so short lived a nuclide and the photon
energy was still too high to provide high resolution images.
Gallium, a known bone-seeker, was being investigated by Hayes and
Edwards for its efficacy as a bone imaging agent when the soft
tumor localizing tendency was observed for carrier-free 67-Ga
citrate (10).

Since that first observation, 67-Ga citrate has been administered to thousands of cancer patients as a diagnostic aid.
Between April 1971 and August 1973, 1022 patient whole body
scintiscan studies were performed by the Nuclear Medicine Department, Clinical Center, National Institutes of Health, on patients
with malignancies (Table 1-1). Selected examples from among these
patients are presented in this monograph. A wide variation in
tumor localization of 67-Ga has been observed with the general
agreement that some tumors consistently concentrate 67-Ga better
than others. The size of the tumor, its localization with respect
to the body surface and to normal bodily sites of 67-Ga concentration,
and the treatment status of the patient have all seemed to be
important considerations in interpreting 67-Ga scintigraphic images.
These variations in 67-Ga concentration from tumor site to tumor
site have resulted in a relatively high rate of false negative
studies. The high potential for false negative findings has placed
emphasis on positive sites of 67-Ga concentration in these studies.
A positive 67-Ga scintigram requires definitive evaluation: a
negative scintigram does not rule out the necessity for further

study.

Chemical and Physical Characteristics

Gallium, like aluminum, is an amphoteric element, behaving
as a metal in acid and as a nonmetal in alkaline media. It has
a blue-gray metallic appearance and may be encountered as liquid
or a solid because of a low melting point (29.8°C). Gallium, with
atomic number 31 and mass numbers 69 and 71 (stable) exists in
three valence states (+1, +2 and +3) (11). The trivalent citrate
compound is used for imaging in nuclear medicine. Attempts at
using other compounds than citrate have encountered problems,
mainly with solubility (12).

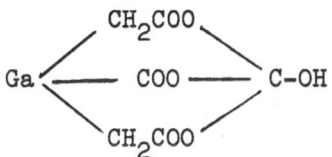

Gallium Citrate

Isotopes of gallium have mass numbers from 64 through 74. Of
these, 67-Ga is the isotope with the best physical characteristics
for scintigraphy at this point in technological development, and is
the one used to perform the studies presented here. Carrier-free
67-Ga is produced in the cyclotron by bombarding a zinc target
with protons. 67-Ga undergoes electron capture decay with a half-
life of 78 hours. Gamma emissions occur between 0.88 and 0.093
MeV with principal photopeaks of 0.093, 0.188, 0.296 and 0.388
MeV.

Imaging Technique

The tendency for 67-Ga to label many types of malignancy and
the metastases of those malignancies has provided a place for this
radionuclide in screening patients with cancer to determine the
extent of the primary tumor and to determine the presence and
location of metastatic lesions. An additional role may be established for 67-Ga in screening patients to help diagnose the presence
or absence of primary malignancy. Since the possibilities are
limitless for sites of cancer involvement, the whole body scan
has become the study of choice when 67-Ga is used as the scanning
agent. Selected adjunctive gamma scintillation camera views can
be helpful in delineating a borderline abnormality and in studying
tumors involving the head and neck, including brain. The gamma
scintillation camera technique is described in Chapter 11.

Whole body scanning with 67-Ga citrate requires 50 µCi/kg of body weight to be given intravenously. After an interval of 48 to 96 hours, the patient returns for whole body scanning. A laxative is given at 12 and at 36 hours before the scan to encourage excretion of stool containing the radionuclide. The patient is made comfortable in the supine position and scanned from head to toe using 5:1 minification without background erase or enhancement. A variety of pulse height window settings are possible. The scans illustrated herein were made with a window from 130 to 330. Generally, the liver count rate is used to determine the intensity. Scanning time varies between 1½ and 2 hours for a person 5'10" tall. Areas of interest are sometimes rescanned with the patient in the lateral position to determine localization of a site in the antero-posterior plane.

The nuclear medical evaluation of patients known to have cancer has frequently required the use of several imaging procedures. The following tests were often ordered for the same patient; liver scintigraphy, brain scintigraphy, whole body skeletal scan and 67-Ga whole body scan. It is advisable to perform the studies in the above mentioned order since it involves the least delay. An initial patient evaluation with 67-Ga will result in interference with other studies and cause a delay (in further scintigraphic studies) for at least one week.

TABLE 1-1

GALLIUM-67 WHOLE BODY SCAN STUDIES
April 1971 - August 1973

Diagnosis	Scans
Lymphomas	178
Hodgkin's Disease	141
Breast Cancers	114
Head and Neck Cancers	97
Malignant Melanoma	92
Leukemia	78
Lung Cancers	65
Central Nervous System Tumors*	27
Primary Bone Cancers	48
Uterine Cancers	43
Soft Tissue Sarcomas	41
Ovarian Carcinomas	9
Pancreatic Cancers	7
Hepatomas	5
Miscellaneous Neoplasms	47
Unknown Malignancies	30

TOTAL 1022**

---

*An additional 60 patients have been studied with brain scintigraphy using the gamma scintillation camera to obtain traditional brain image views.

**This figure represents patient studies with a whole body anterior and posterior view per study. Additional views including lateral views and repeat partial or total whole body views are not included in this number.

CHAPTER 2

Metabolism

Louis G. Gelrud, M. D. and James C. Arseneau, M. D.[*]

Section on Diseases of the Liver, Metabolic Diseases
Branch, National Institute of Arthritis, Metabolism
and Digestive Diseases

and

[*] Medicine Branch, National Cancer Institute

National Institutes of Health, Bethesda, Maryland

A detailed study of 67-Ga distribution in humans (24) has been
performed, showing that the majority of the isotope 67-Ga is bound
to plasma transferrin, haptoglobin and albumin (65) following the
intravenous injection of carrier free 67-Ga citrate (30,31). Over
the 24 hours after injection, the kidney excretes 12% of the administered dose and contains the highest concentration of 67-Ga.
After the first day, the liver becomes the major route of excretion.
Between 48 and 72 hours, the usual scanning period, the highest
concentrations are seen in the bones, liver and spleen. In the
first week, about 1/3 of the administered dose of the isotope is
excreted, and the remaining 2/3 is distributed within the liver
(6%), spleen (1%), kidney (2%), skeleton including marrow (24%),
and other soft tissues (34%) (16). Other organs with relatively
high concentration include the adrenals, bowel and lung. Localization within mammary tissue during lactation has been reported (35)
(Fig. 2-1) and a physiologically variable and unexplained mammary
localization has also been observed in nonlactating patients
(Fig. 3-5). The lacrimal glands may also be variably observed.

In studies at NIH (25), serial whole body counting and blood
plasma retention curves of 67-Ga activity in patients dosed with
this nuclide for whole body scanning have suggested accumulation
of activity in the cellular fraction of blood in chronic myelogenous leukemia (CML) patients with high leukocyte counts.

7

Patients with normal leukocyte counts and one patient with a marked
elevation of lymphocytes and circulating lymphosarcoma cells did not
show any marked cellular accumulation of 67-Ga. In vivo and in
vitro studies of the uptake of 67-Ga by whole blood revealed
accumulation of activity mainly in the leukocyte fraction (15).
A small amount of 67-Ga activity was also associated with erythro-
cytes, and appeared to be mainly bound to the RBC membrane. In
vitro studies of 67-Ga uptake by mouse and human bone marrow and
human peripheral blood revealed uptake primarily in the granulocytic fraction. No uptake by lymphocytes was demonstrated. In
the mouse marrow, 67-Ga uptake was seen exclusively in the mature
granulocyte fraction with primarily cytoplasmic localization.
Several patients with CML have received whole body 67-Ga scans
which show increased activity in the areas of leukemic infiltra-
tions. In vitro studies of 67-Ga uptake by granulocytes suggest
that this increased activity is more related to the absolute
number of cells, rather than to an increased affinity for 67-Ga by
CML leukocytes.

The concentration of the isotope within malignancies appears
to vary with extent of tumor viability. Living cells concentrate
more 67-Ga than necrotic tissue, while fibrotic tissue concentrates
an intermediate amount (18). If the neoplasm is treated with
either cytotoxic drugs or radiation therapy, a diminution and then
a cessation of 67-Ga localization is observed (13,19,20). Autoradiographs of 67-Ga labelled tumor cells examined by light microscope have been interpreted as showing cytoplasmic localization
(21). Subcellular fractionation has demonstrated that the majority
of the radioactivity is associated with a lysosome-rich supernatant
(22). Further, autoradiographs studied by electron microscope have
localized the isotope to electron-dense, single-membrane bound
subcellular organelles which are typical of lysosomes (23). The
evidence to date suggests that the binding site within neoplastic
cells may be the lysosome itself.

Inflammatory lesions have also been visualized following
67-Ga injection, and localization has been reported in a wide
range of inflammatory states (25,29). Pyogenic lesions such as
bacterial pneumonia and abscess, as well as active granulomatous
lesions such as tuberculosis and sarcoidosis, have been observed
to concentrate the isotope. The intensity and visualization of
inflammatory lesions appears to correlate with the activity of
the underlying inflammatory response. Healed or inactive lesions
fail to show uptake of 67-Ga while active lesions show intense
concentration of the isotope (28). Effective therapy of the
underlying cause of inflammation has resulted in a gradual diminution and eventual disappearance of 67-Ga activity from the area
of the lesion (29).

The inflammatory response to an inciting stimulus consists basically of an increased vascular permeability and an influx and accumulation of granulocytes. 67-Ga concentration within inflammatory lesions has been demonstrated experimentally (25,28,32) and clinically (16,20,28,29). When the time course of 67-Ga localization within experimental inflammatory lesions is observed, older lesions with a decreased vascular permeability are found to have the same visual time course of localization as less mature lesions with an increased vascular permeability (33). The uptake of 67-Ga in inflammatory lesions seems to correlate best with the presence or formation of a granulocytic mass capable of binding the radio-isotope (15). When experimental abscesses were produced in the limbs of leukopenic animals and the time course of 67-Ga incorporation into the lesions observed, a delay in 67-Ga uptake was seen in those partially leukopenic and a complete abolition of 67-Ga uptake into the abscesses was observed in the almost totally leukopenic animals (33). These findings would indicate that changes in vascular permeability are probably important in the initial delivery of 67-Ga to an inflammatory site, but the appearance and accumulation of lysosome rich granulocytes at the site of the inflammatory lesion coincided with the binding of 67-Ga.

The radionuclide 67-Ga has attracted interest because of its ability to localize in and allow scintigraphic visualization of various malignancies (10,17,18). In addition, the isotope has the capability of localizing within inflammatory lesions. The uptake of the isotope by both neoplastic and inflammatory lesions appears to correlate with the underlying viability of the pathologic process since effective therapy causes a diminution in 67-Ga localization in both types of lesion. Available evidence seems to indicate that the subcellular binding site for 67-Ga in these abnormal cells is the lysosome. The mechanism of 67-Ga accumulation appears to be diffusion into the cells with binding and retention in those with lysosomes, or with lysosome-like granules.

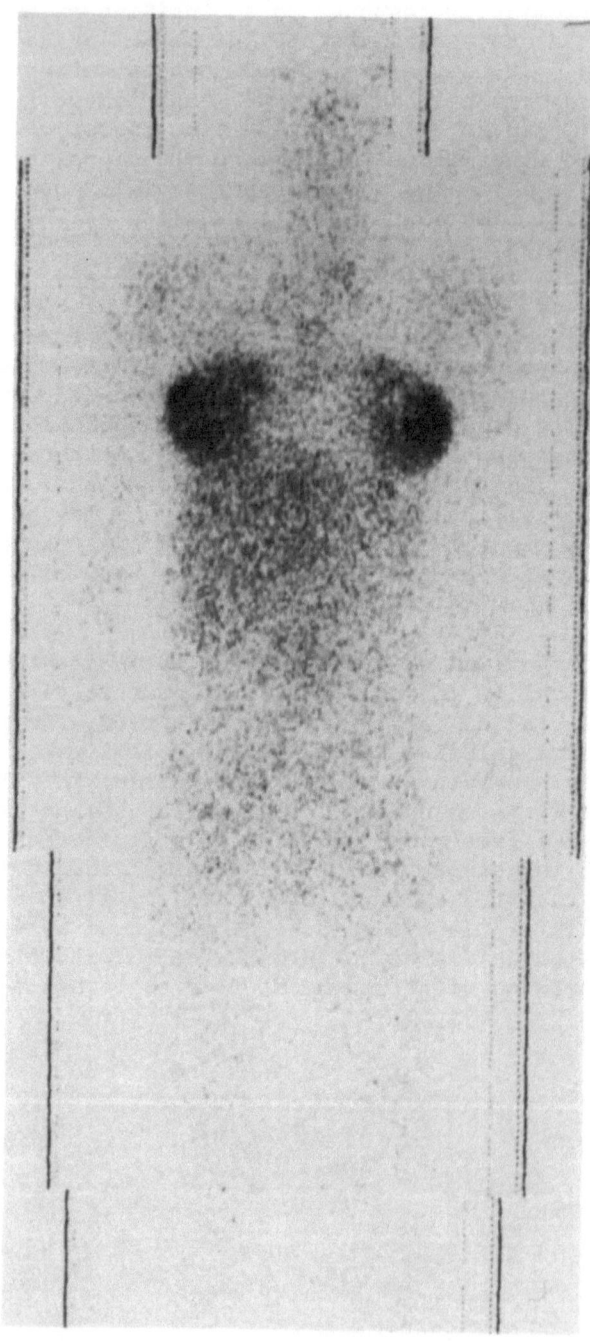

Fig. 2-1. Localization of 67-Ga in both breasts of a postpartum patient with Hodgkin's disease. Hormones had not been administered to suppress lactation.

CHAPTER 3

Scintigraphic Interpretation

Michael S. Milder, M. D.

Department of Nuclear Medicine, Clinical Center

National Institutes of Health, Bethesda, Maryland

The varying affinity of 67-Ga for different tissues results in a nonuniform distribution in the body. This distribution yields a photoscan showing greater activity over certain organs such as bones and liver, than in the rest of the body. In addition, normal changes in the metabolic activity of these organs can produce further alterations in the scan appearance. Because of these many variables, accurate interpretation of the 67-Ga study requires familiarity with the wide range of normal scan patterns.

The results of 67-Ga scintigraphy in a series of normal volunteers have never been described. Our knowledge of normal 67-Ga localization comes from observation of uninvolved areas in patients studied because of neoplastic disease. These findings have been fairly consistent in studies involving hundreds of patients and several groups of investigators (17,34,69). The following summary of the normal 67-Ga scan appearance is based on such observations in cancer patients. Examples of normal whole body rectilinear scans are shown in Figs. 3-1A and B and 3-2A and B, demonstrating the range of variation in bone and soft tissue uptake.

Head and Neck: Figure 3-1A shows the normal distribution of 67-Ga activity concentrated in the osseous structures of the skull, and in the region of the lacrimal glands and the nasopharynx (See Fig. 11-1). Nasopharyngeal activity is usually the most prominent feature of the scan in the head and neck. This probably results from uptake in the lymphoid tissue of Waldeyer's ring. Because of its prominence, normal uptake can make the diagnosis of pathological lesions in the nasopharynx very difficult. For example, it is difficult to distinguish the midline granuloma in Fig. 3-3 from normal activity.

11

Accumulation of the 67-Ga in the lacrimal and salivary glands is quite variable. The factors influencing this uptake are not known. However, in some patients normal concentration of 67-Ga in the salivary glands may be quite prominent (Figs. 6-1 and 6-2). Interpretation of high cervical activity must be done with caution because it is difficult to differentiate submaxillary gland uptake from neoplastic lymph nodes. This requires correlation with the history and physical examination. Non-neoplastic nodes rarely accumulate 67-Ga.

Thorax: In the thorax, 67-Ga is normally distributed within the ribs, sternum, clavicles, spine and scapulae (Fig. 2A and B). These structures may occasionally cause a problem of interpretation.

On the anterior view, concentration of 67-Ga in the sternum may be so prominent as to mimic tumor uptake. The triangular shape of the manubrium with the apex pointed downward and the superior orientation are of some benefit in differentiating the sternum from enlarged hilar or peritracheal lymph nodes. These structures can be separated by a lateral view of the chest.

On the posterior view, the lower ends of the scapulae nearly always show a prominent concentration near the lateral chest wall. This must be differentiated from rib lesions and tumor in axillary or lateral thoracic nodes (Fig. 3-5A and B). Again lateral views may be of help.

There is occasional uptake in the breasts which is particularly prominent under the physiologic stimulus of the menarche, cyclic estrogenic and progestational agents, or pregnancy (35) (See Fig. 2-1). Fig. 3-6 is an example of accentuated breast uptake associated with oral contraceptives. Note that this activity is diffuse and bilaterally symmetrical.

The breast is also a common site of myeloblastomas, which may mimic physiologic uptake in leukemia patients. In such cases the uptake is usually more focal and asymmetrical.

Abdomen: 67-Ga is normally concentrated within the liver and spleen, but other intraabdominal structures are normally not seen (Fig. 3-1A and B). On the posterior view the spine and sacrum are prominent.

The most common problem of photoscan interpretation in the abdomen is the presence of 67-Ga within the bowel. Usually this appears in a linear pattern in the region of all or part of the colon and is easily recognizable. Occasionally intestinal accumulation will simulate focal mass lesions (Fig. 3-7A). Correct interpretation is then impossible unless abdominal views are repeated after further purging the bowel (Fig. 3-7B).

Liver uptake is usually a conspicuous feature of anterior and posterior 67-Ga images. The concentration may vary from one study to the next due to unknown factors. A tumor with a low level of 67-Ga uptake may be hidden within the liver (Fig. 3-8A) but may be visualized in other areas against a lower background activity. While most hepatomas exhibit some 67-Ga affinity, not all will exceed the liver activity to become visible on the scan (56). "Cold" areas on the 67-Ga liver scan usually indicate benign tumors, cysts, or radiation therapy fields (36).

The kidneys have the greatest activity in the body in the first day after the intravenous dose of 67-Ga, but by the time of scanning the concentration has usually fallen greatly. Hayes has demonstrated excellent visualization of the kidneys in a rat scanned at one hour with 67-Ga (7). However, the kidneys do not normally appear on the 48-72 hour scan in man. Definite renal activity on the scan should suggest any one of the following: scanning too soon after administration of 67-Ga; neoplastic involvement of the kidneys; pyelonephritis; or obstructive renal disease (Fig. 3-9A and B).

Pelvis: The pelvis is often difficult to interpret because of residual feces in the rectum and the large amount of bone uptake. Activity is usually prominent in the sacrum and around the hip joints with uptake also in the ilia and ischia. The scrotum and vagina often show some uptake of 67-Ga, the mechanism of which is unknown. The bladder does not contain 67-Ga activity. Because of the high pelvic concentration of 67-Ga, interpretation and detection of neoplasia has been least reliable in this area.

Extremities: The normal 67-Ga study shows no definite activity within the long bones of the extremities, but a diffuse increase in uptake is usually present around the large joints; shoulders, elbows, hips, and knees. In certain physiologic and pathologic conditions the localization in the extremities may be markedly increased. This is a normal finding in children with rapidly growing bones. The increased uptake is usually confined to the ends of the long bones (Fig. 3-10). Physical stress may also cause increased uptake, also probably due to augmented bone turnover. This may be observed in people with hemiplegia or amputation (Fig. 3-1). Accentuation of the diaphyseal as well as the epiphyseal parts of the bones is a frequent finding in leukemia (38). This is most pronounced in blast crisis of chronic myelogenous leukemia (Fig. 3-2A and B). In other malignancies increased bone uptake is occasionally seen without evidence of bone or marrow invasion. This finding must therefore not be considered diagnostic of bone involvement in all patients. Decreased bone uptake in an area may result from disease or previous irradiation.

Residual 67-Ga at the injection site may give a focus of
activity in the extremities (Fig. 5-4B). The site of injection
should be noted at the time of the study.

Lymph Nodes: Lymph nodes are the first site to which most
tumors metastasize. They are the most frequently observed abnormal
structures on a 67-Ga study. The visualization of lymph nodes on
a 67-Ga scan is always pathological. Lymph node uptake in reactive
hyperplasia or infectious mononucleosis has not been reported.
Thus, the node-bearing areas are visualized only when involved by
tumor or abscess.

Familiarity with the distribution of the lymph node groups
on the 67-Ga scan facilitates recognition of metastatic disease.
The major lymph node groups are demonstrated on the scan in Figs.
3-12A and B in a patient with widespread Hodgkin's disease. Notice
that the para-aortic nodes are seen best on the anterior view because
they enlarge anteriorly. These nodes are located at either side
of the midline and are oriented along a vertical midline axis.
In contrast, 67-Ga in the bowel is usually seen laterally and
crosses the midline on a horizontal axis. The iliac nodes spread
laterally and may be confused with 67-Ga in the cecum or sigmoid
colon.

The technique of whole body rectilinear scanning has been
suitable for screening for metastatic disease. In an area such as
the head and neck, where there may be difficulty in interpreting
the rectilinear study, additional gamma camera views have been
helpful.

It has proven useful to obtain whole body rectilinear bone
scans prior to the 67-Ga study. Bone scans have aided the subsequent interpretation of whole body 67-Ga scans.

Other organ scans such as brain and liver, obtained prior
to the 67-Ga study, should be reviewed at the time of interpretation
of the whole body 67-Ga scans.

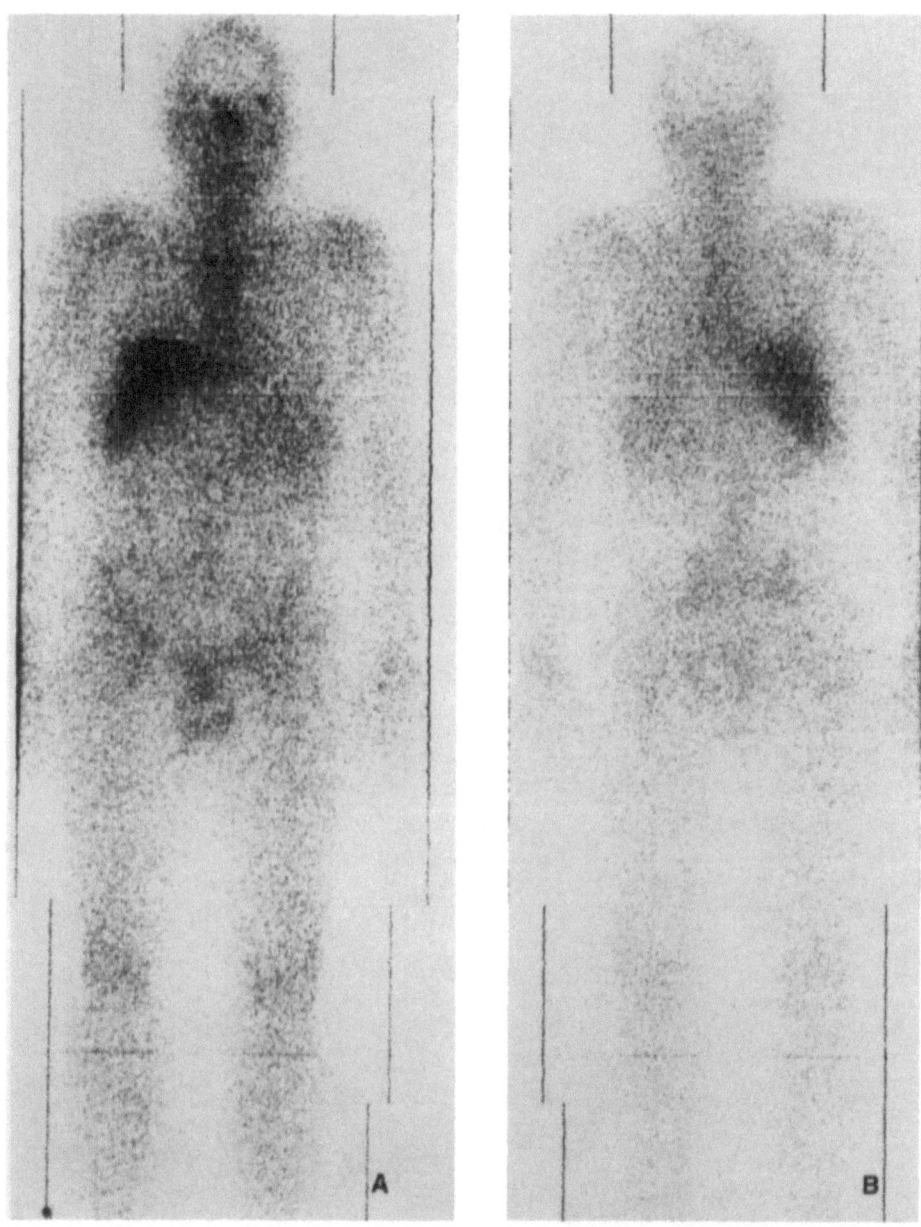

Fig. 3-1. Normal anterior (A) and posterior (B) rectilinear scans
with 67-Ga in a 54-year-old man with history of histiocytic lymphoma. There is normal accumulation in the region of the orbits,
nasopharynx, liver, spleen, pelvic bones and genitalia on the
anterior view. The posterior view shows the spine and sacrum in
addition. There is moderate background activity in the soft
tissues.

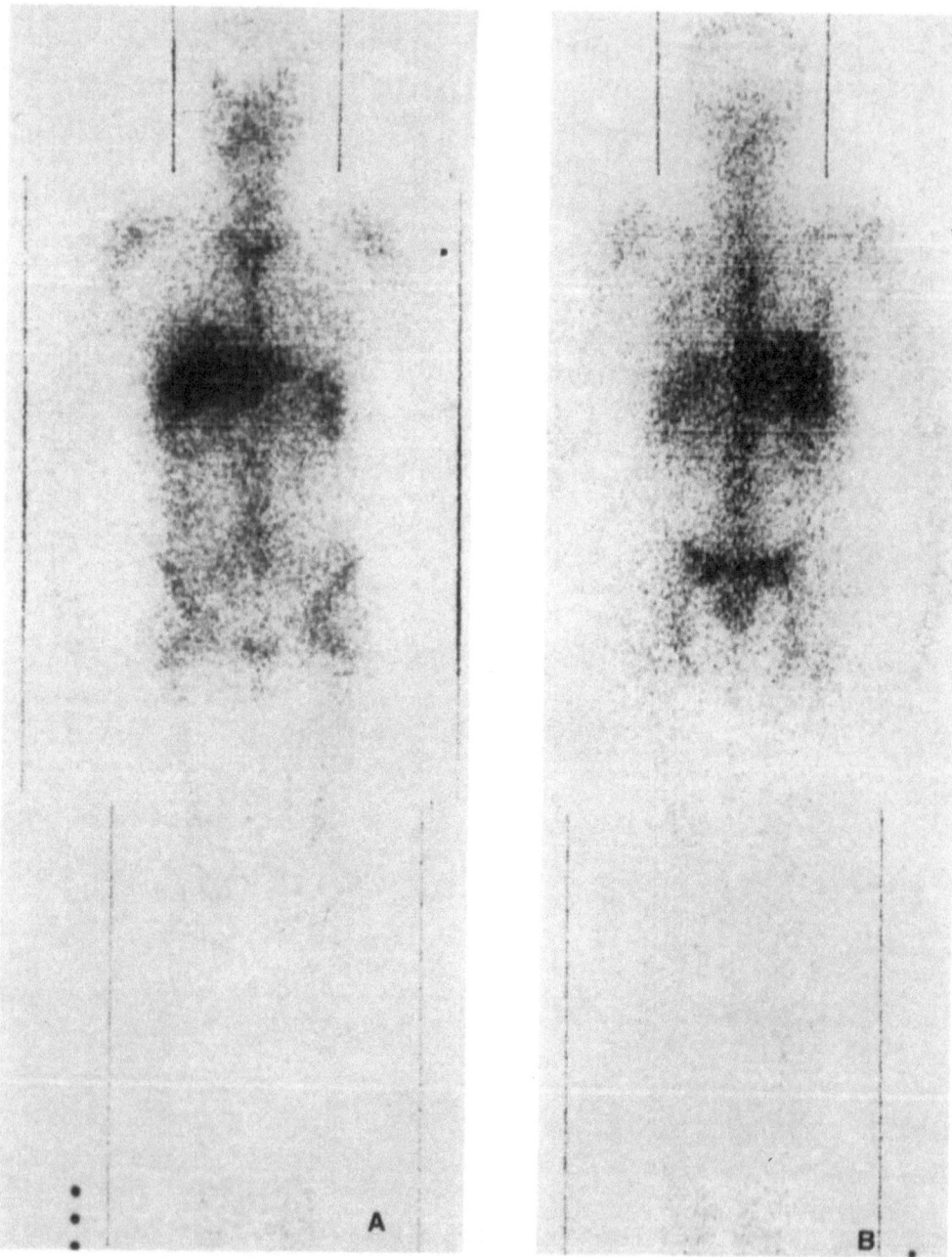

Fig. 3-2. Normal anterior (A) and posterior (B) scans with 67-Ga in a 44-year-old woman with cancer of the cervix. In comparison with Fig. 1 there is less tissue background and greater concentration in the bones, showing clearly the sternum, proximal humerus and femur, scapular tips, spine and pelvic girdle.

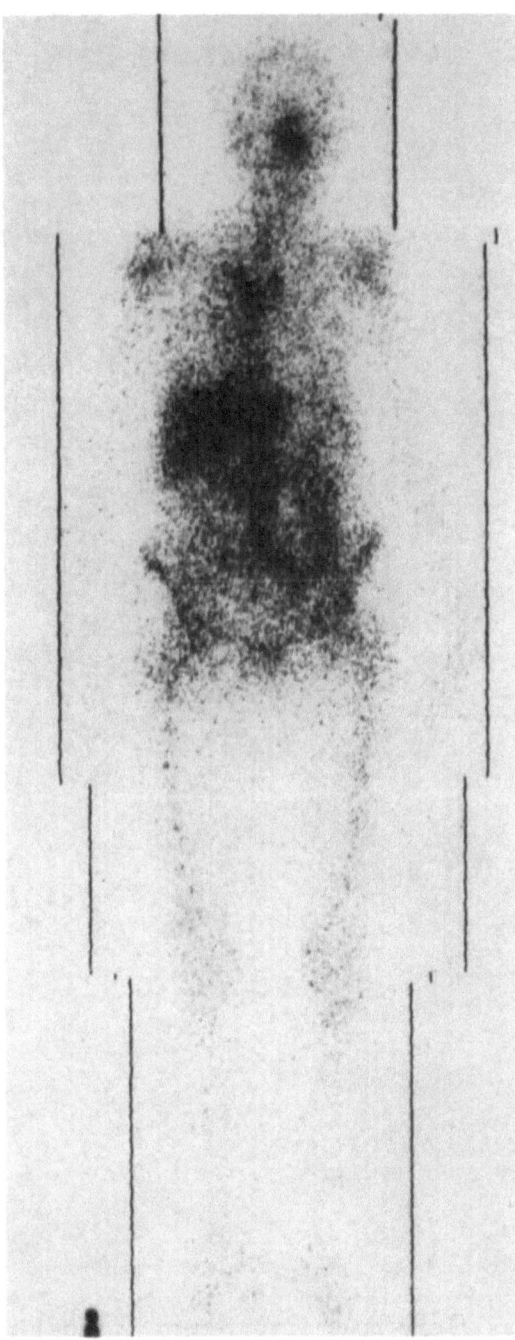

Fig. 3-3. Nasopharyngeal lesions are difficult to distinguish from normal 67-Ga concentration. Anterior scan shows prominent nasal uptake in a woman with lethal midline granuloma.

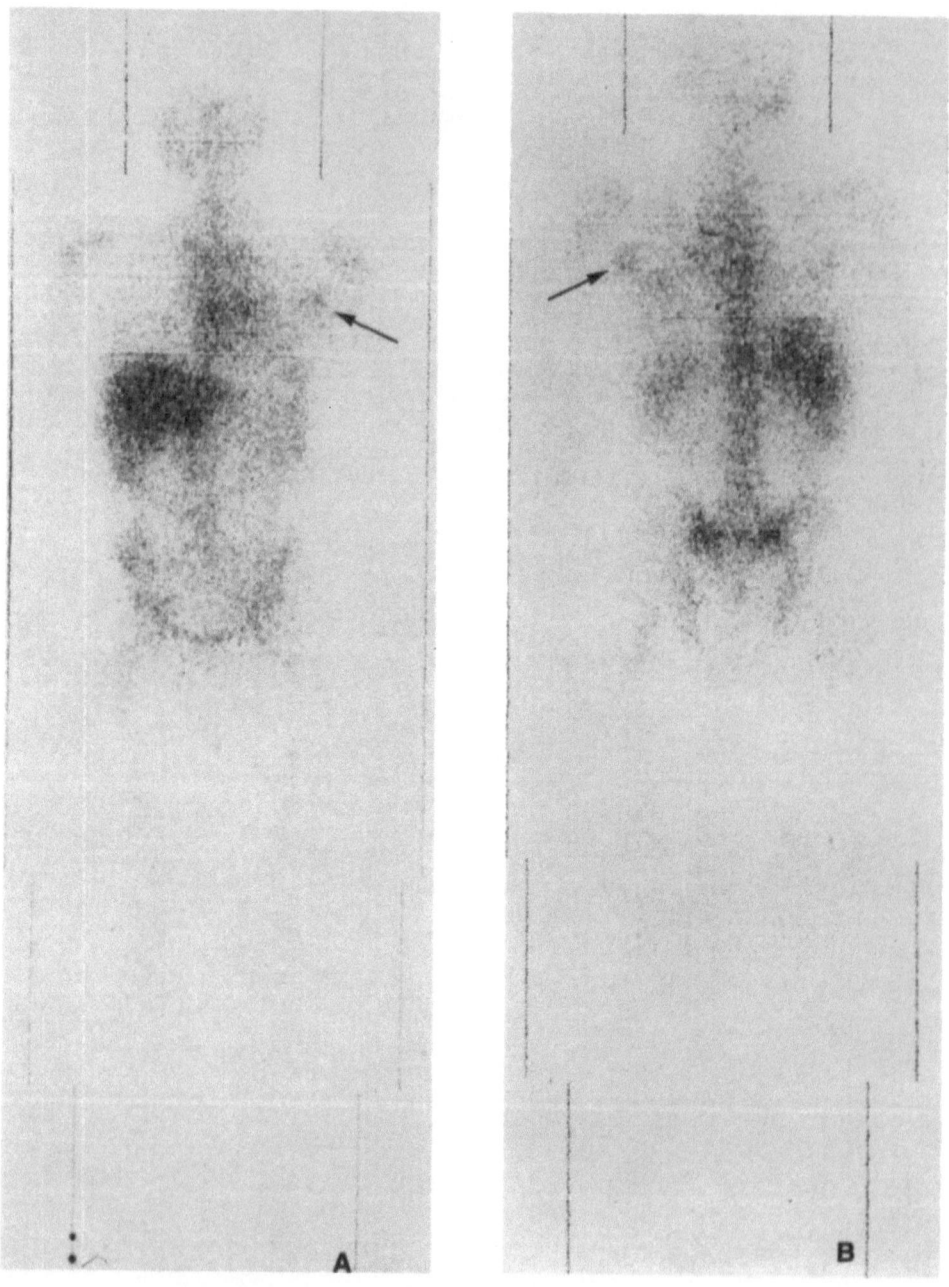

Fig. 3-4. Left axillary node involvement (arrow) in a 49-year-old man with untreated stage III Hodgkin's disease. This must be distinguished from normal uptake in the nearby scapular tips seen bilaterally. The axillary nodes may be seen anteriorly (A) as well as posteriorly (B).

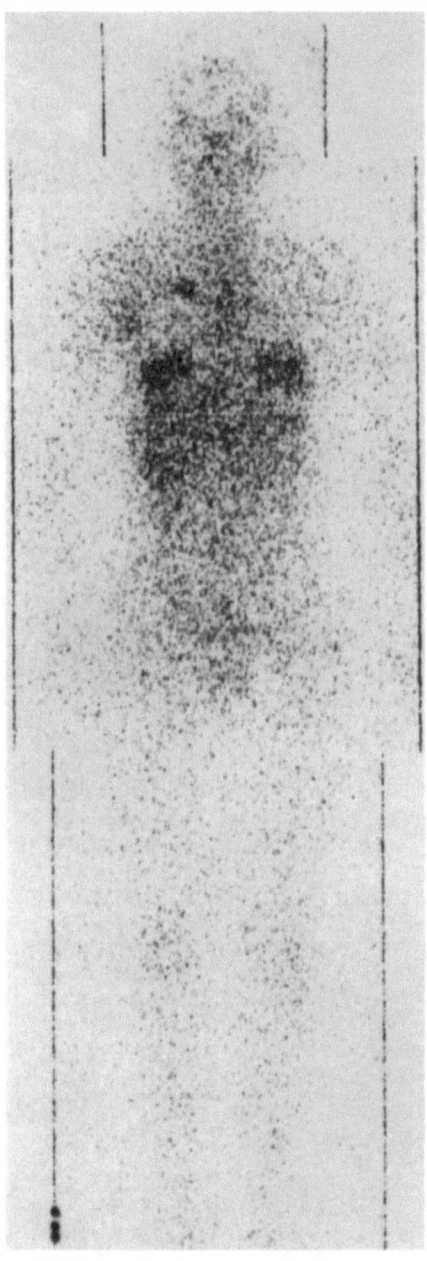

Fig. 3-5. Bilateral breast uptake seen in a 26-year-old woman with stage IV Hodgkin's disease. The breasts were normal on examination and the patient was not, and had not been pregnant. She was receiving a number of medications, including vinblastine and oral contraceptives. (Note abnormalities in right axilla and right chest.)

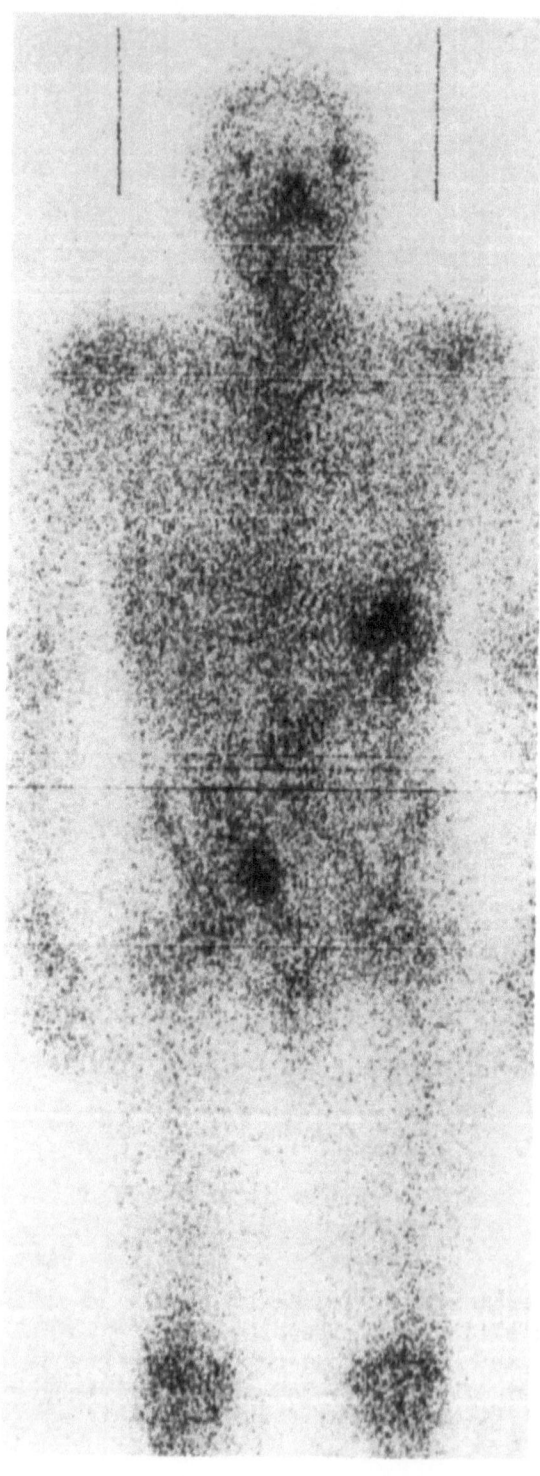

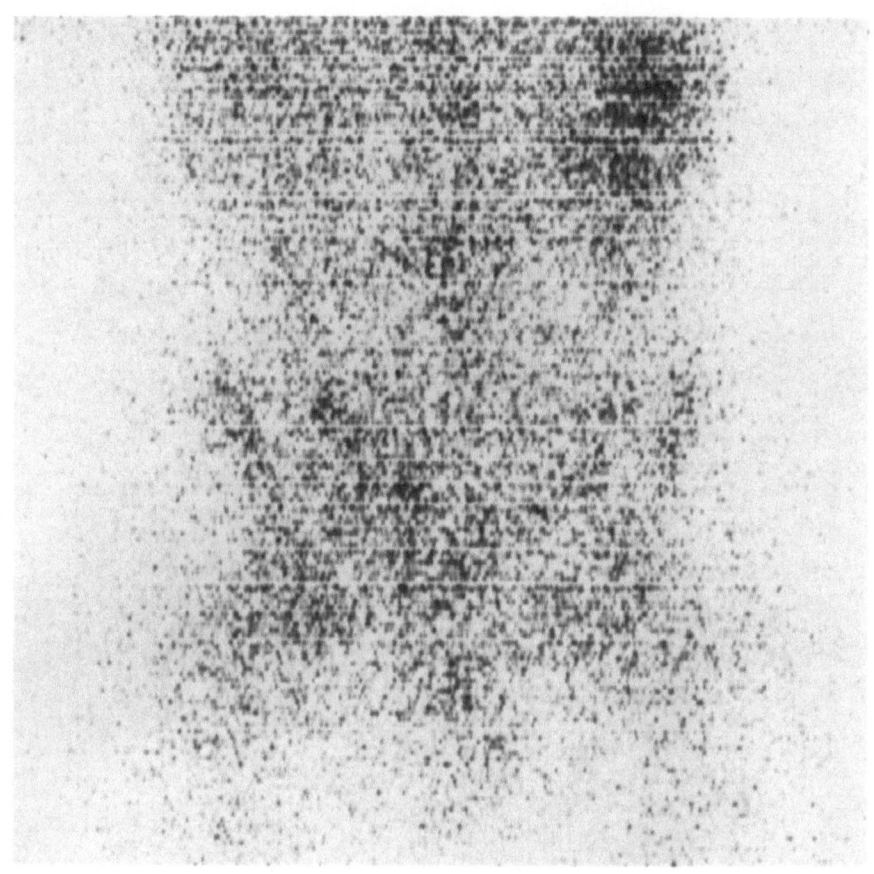

Fig. 3-6. 67-Ga accumulation in bowel contents in a 48-year-old man with chronic myelogenous leukemia. (A) The 48-hour anterior view after inadequate bowel cleansing shows focal accumulation in the cecum and splenic flexure joined by linear activity in the ascending and transverse colon. (B) Twenty-four hours later, after further cathartics, the abdomen has changed in appearance with breaking and partial clearing up of the fecal masses and movement into the descending colon. This change supported the conclusion that the abdominal activity was fecal and within the bowel lumen.

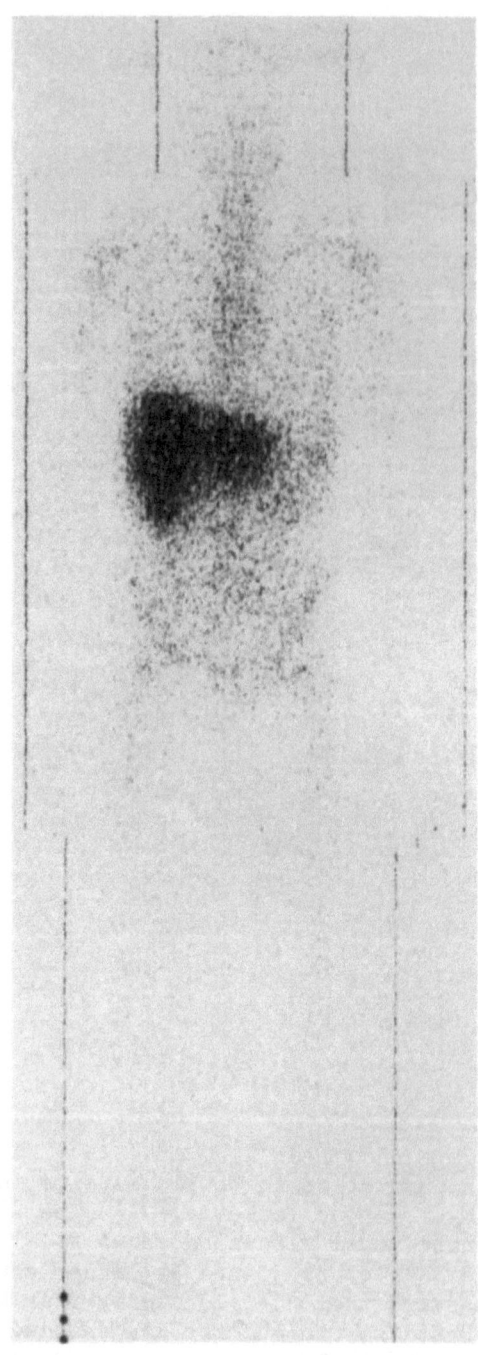

Fig. 3-7A. Hepatic metastases in a 49-year-old man with malignant melanoma: The 67-Ga scan shows uniform uptake by normal liver and tumor, making liver metastases inapparent (see Fig. 3-7B).

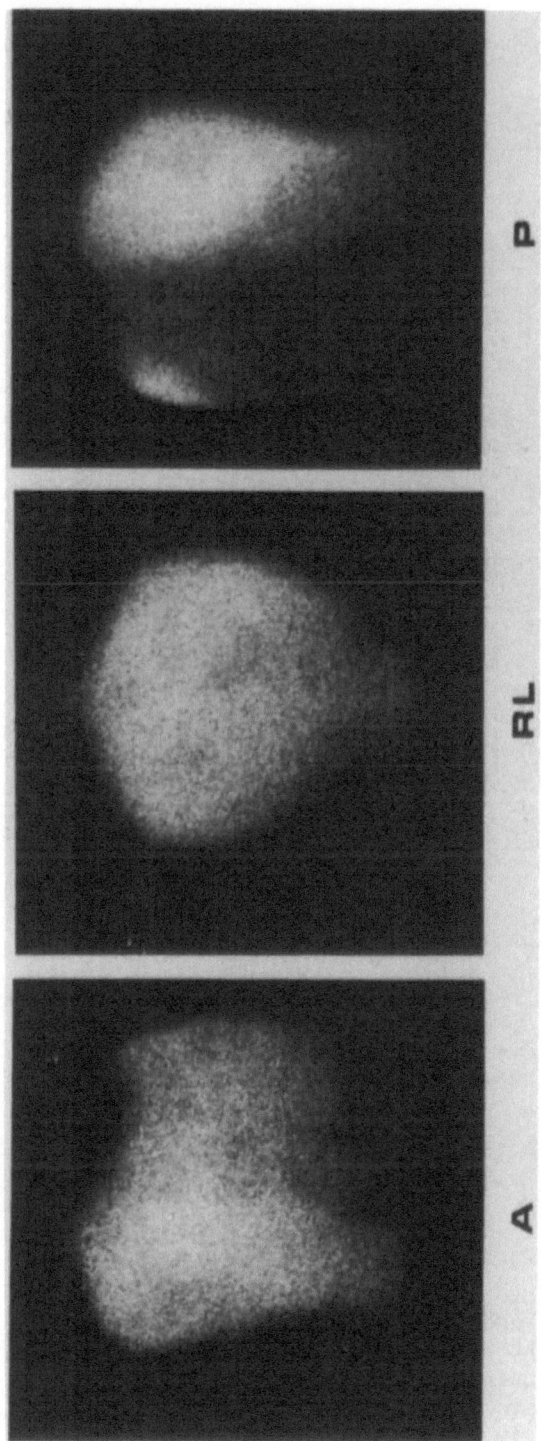

Fig. 3-7B. Hepatic metastases in a 49-year-old man with malignant melanoma (continued): A 99m-Tc sulfur colloid liver scan shows "cold" areas on the anterior, right lateral and posterior views. The abnormality of 99m-Tc sulfur colloid scan was supported by markedly deteriorating liver function tests. A = anterior; RL = right lateral; P = posterior.

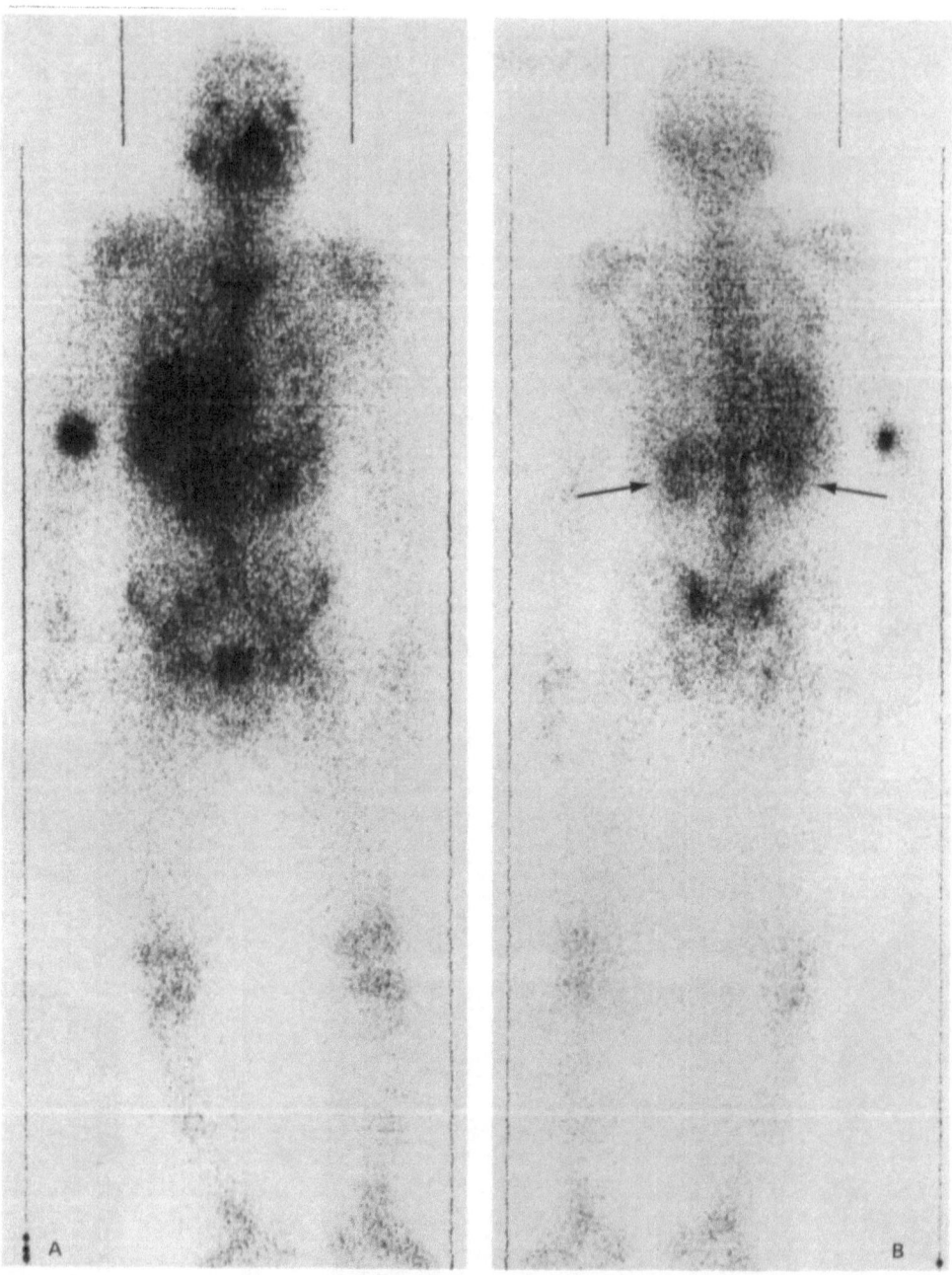

Fig. 3-8. Kidney uptake, anterior (A) and posterior (B) in a
19-year-old male with acute myelocytic leukemia. The patient had
terminal candida septicemia and acute tubular necrosis. Note that
the right kidney image is contiguous with the inferior liver
margin.

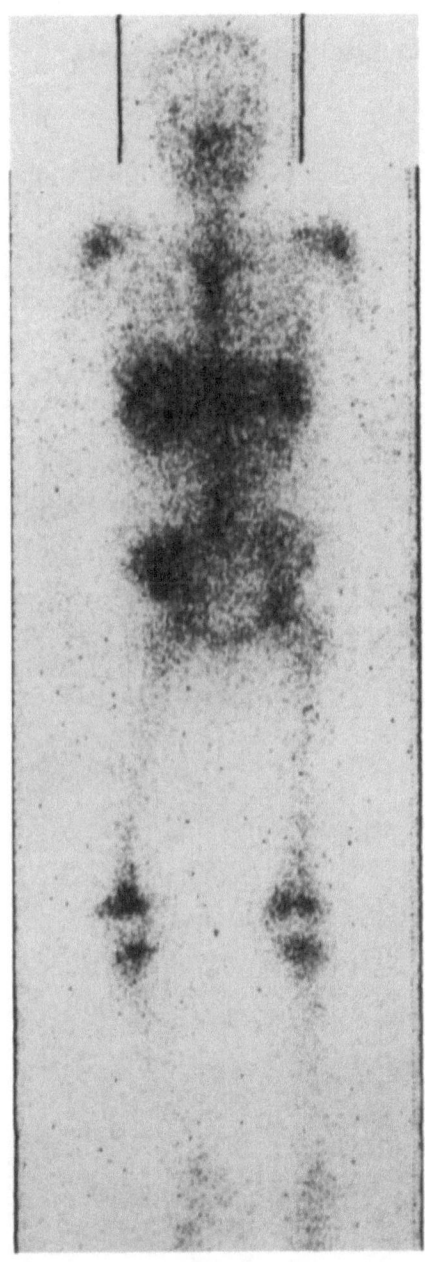

Fig. 3-9. Bone uptake in an adolescent patient is greater than that in the usual adult patient. This anterior 67-Ga scan shows prominent activity in the ends of the long bones in a 12-year-old girl with Ewing's sarcoma of the right ilium. With the exception of the 67-Ga concentration in the right ilium, the bone uptake is normal for this age group.

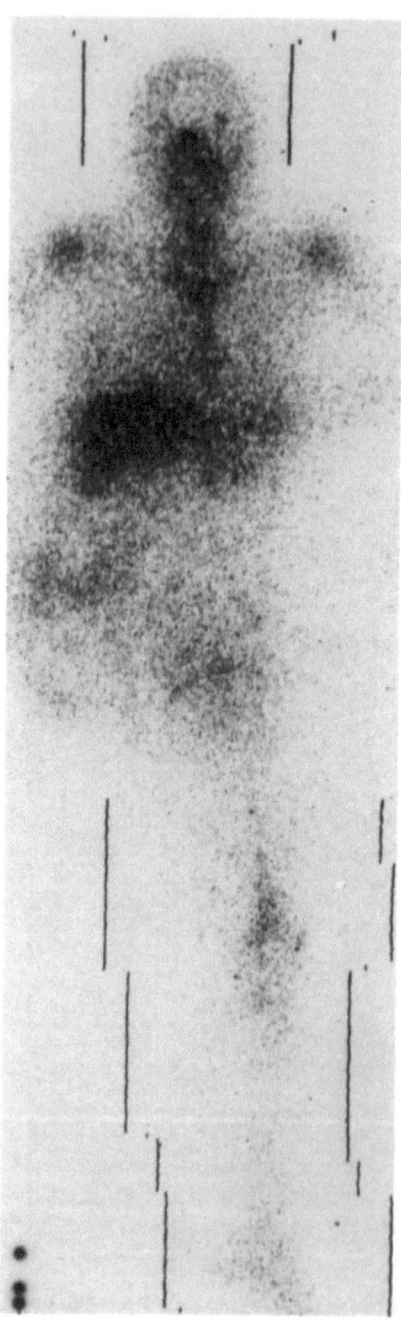

Fig. 3-10.   Increased bone uptake due to weight-bearing in a
46-year-old woman nine years following hemipelvectomy for stage IV
cancer of the cervix.   Accentuated activity is seen in the lower
end of the femur.

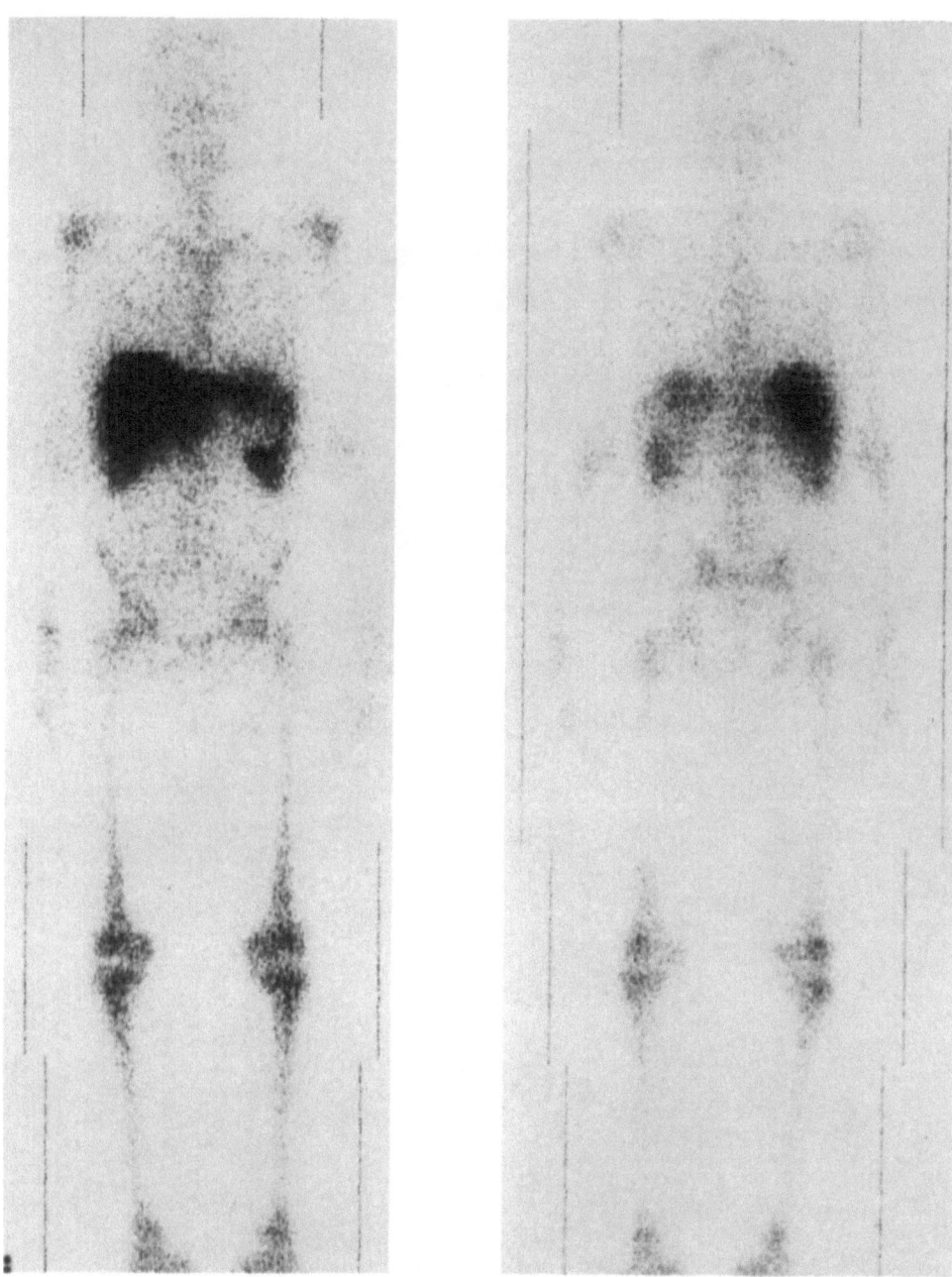

Fig. 3-11. Increased bone uptake in a 61-year-old man with chronic myelogenous leukemia in blast crisis. Bone activity extends throughout the shafts of the long bones. Note the infarct in the midportion of the spleen seen on the anterior (A) and posterior (B) views.

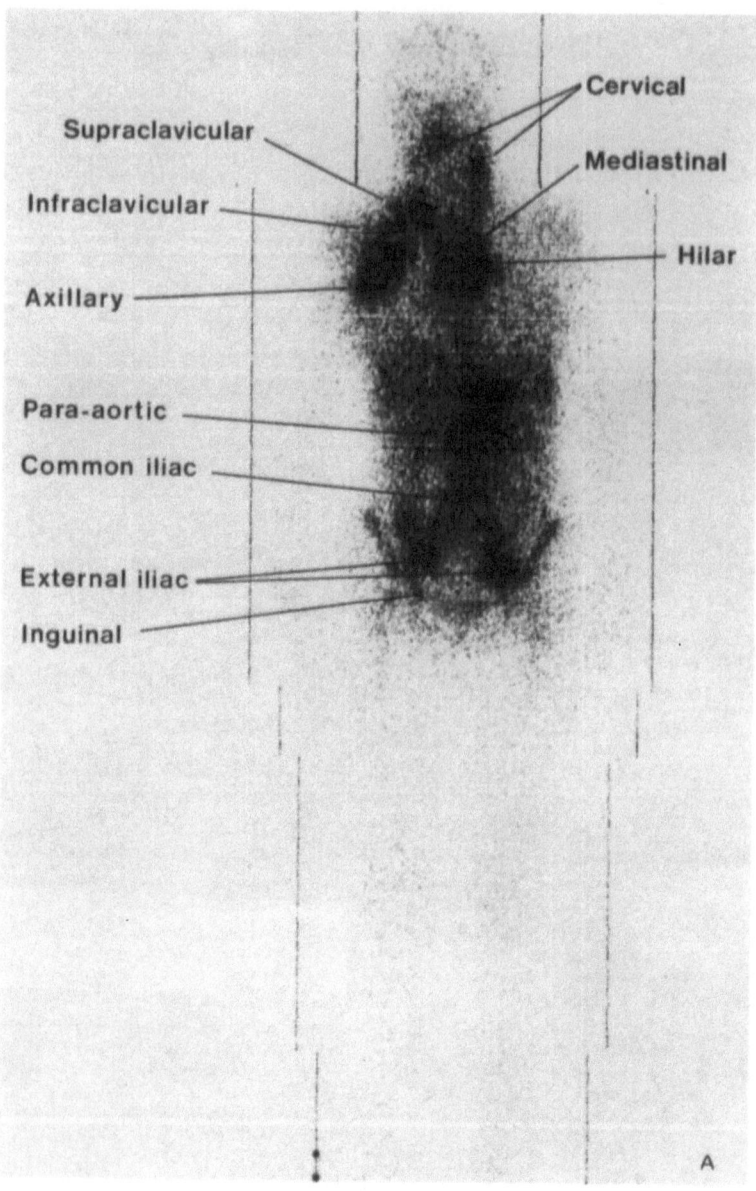

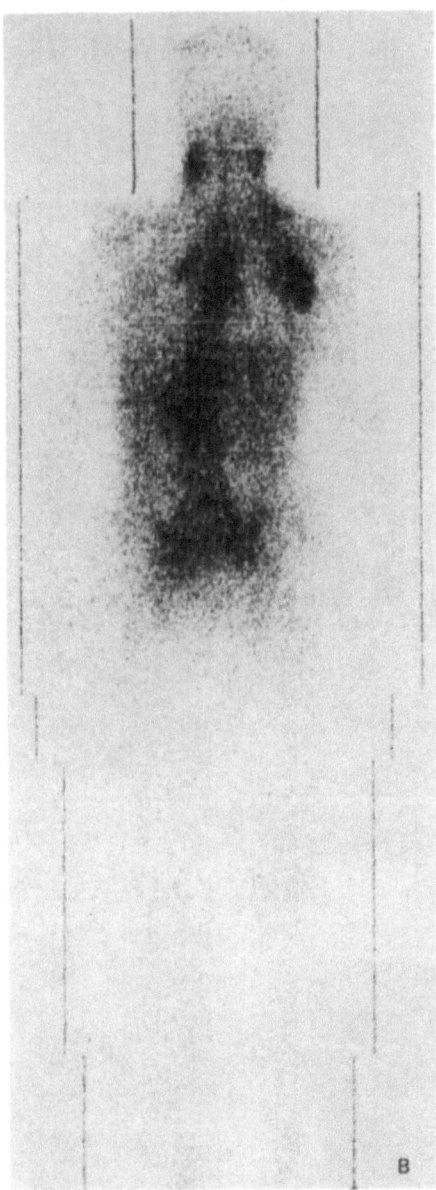

Fig. 3-12. Location of major lymph node groups in a 25-year-old woman with stage III Hodgkin's disease. Lymph node groups are labelled on the anterior scan (A) and can be compared with their appearance on the posterior view (B). The patient had palpable adenopathy in the right and left cervical chains, the right supra-clavicular, right axillary and right inguinal nodes. She had definite radiologic evidence of tumor in the anterior mediastinum, the paraaortic nodes, and bilateral iliac nodes.

CHAPTER 4

Bone Tumors

Robert S. Frankel, M. D.

Department of Nuclear Medicine, Clinical Center

National Institutes of Health, Bethesda, Maryland

Although 67-Ga is generally recognized for its localization in metastases to soft tissue, it is often seen to detect skeletal lesions as well. Because of this propensity for bone lesions, 67-Ga scintigraphy may be used in conjunction with bone scintigraphy to enhance the diagnostic capability of either method used alone.

Primary skeletal tumors which have been studied with 67-Ga citrate scintigraphy include Ewing's sarcoma, osteogenic sarcoma, fibrosarcoma, chondrosarcoma, and other undifferentiated bone sarcomas. A large series of patients with Ewing's sarcoma was studied at the National Institutes of Health. The detection of the Ewing's primary tumor by 67-Ga scintigraphy was as effective as skeletal scanning and diagnostic roentgenography. This has generally been the case in other primary bone malignancies as well. 67-Ga scintigraphy, however, may be more valuable than routine skeletal scintigraphy in determining the extent of involvement by the primary tumor since many primary bone malignancies have accompanying soft tissue involvement which will be demonstrated by 67-Ga scanning but not by bone scanning.

67-Ga scintigraphy has been more accurate in detecting skeletal metastases from primary bone tumors than roentgenography but not as accurate as skeletal scintigraphy. Lung metastases are particularly frequent in Ewing's sarcoma and osteogenic sarcoma and are detected far more efficiently by chest roentgenography than by 67-Ga scintigraphy. On the other hand, bone tumors metastasizing to the mediastinum or retroperitoneum although rare, are detected with greater efficiency on 67-Ga scans than by radiographic studies.

31

    In summary, the use of 67-Ga rectilinear scintigraphy appears
to be of advantage mainly for the detection of metastases from
primary bone tumors to soft tissue other than the lung. The technique is less accurate than 99m-Tc polyphosphate rectilinear
scintigraphy in the detection of skeletal metastases from primary
bone tumors.

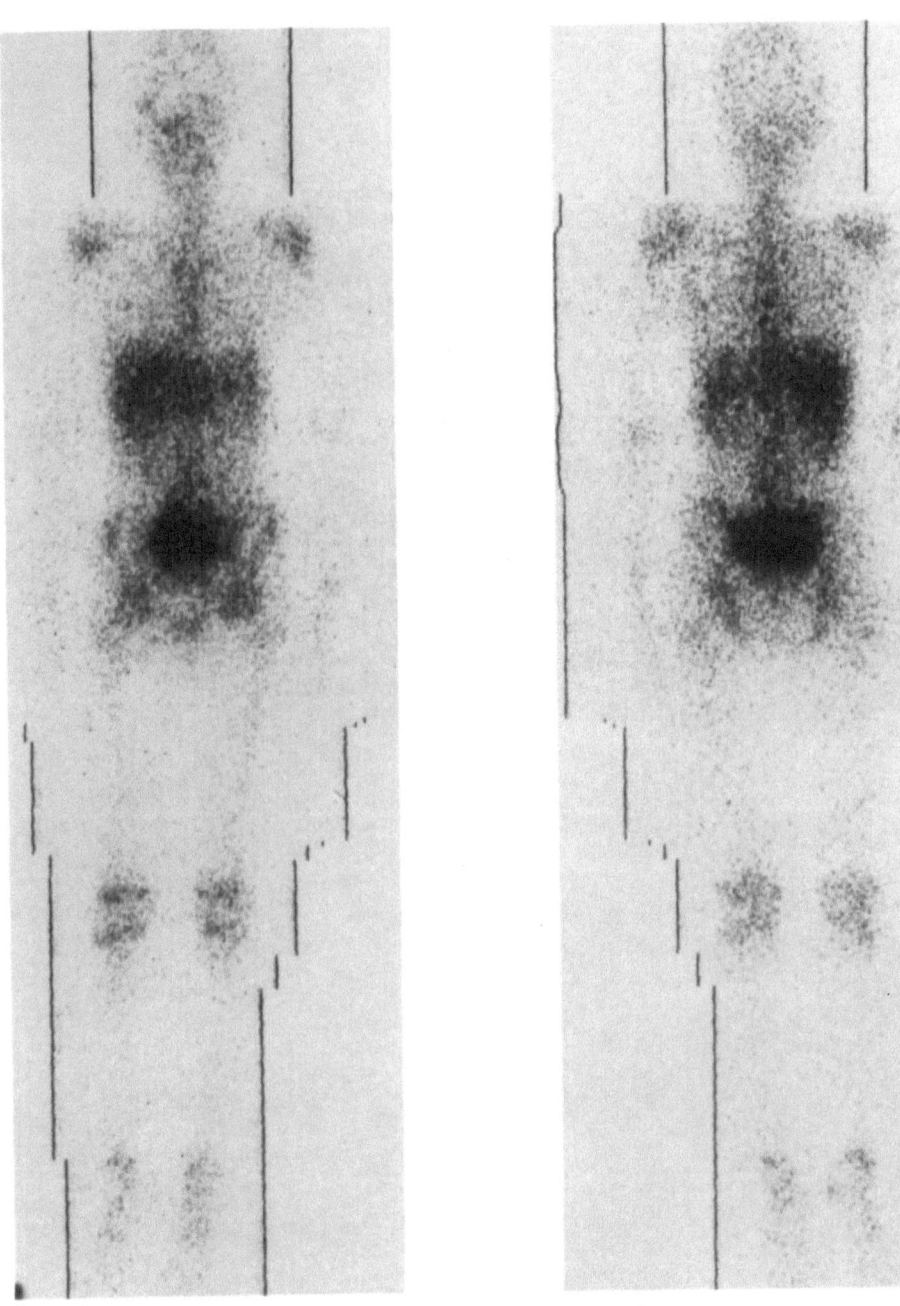

Fig. 4-1. Anterior and posterior whole body scans of a 14-year-old girl showing a large area of increased 67-Ga accumulation in the region of the sacrum. Roentgenograms showed a sclerotic lesion of the sacrum. Biopsy revealed osteogenic sarcoma. The patient received palliative chemotherapy.

Fig. 4-2. Fifteen-year-old girl with a
proven osteogenic sarcoma of the left
shoulder. Anterior whole body 67-Ga
scintigram shows abnormal nuclide accumulation at the site of the patient's
primary tumor. No other abnormalities
are present.

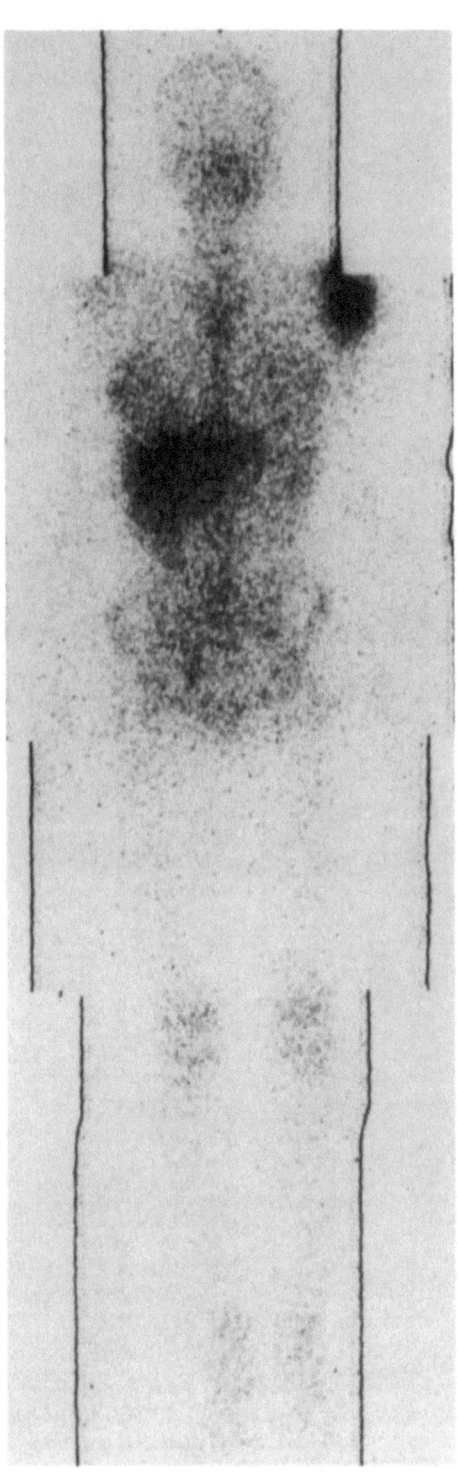

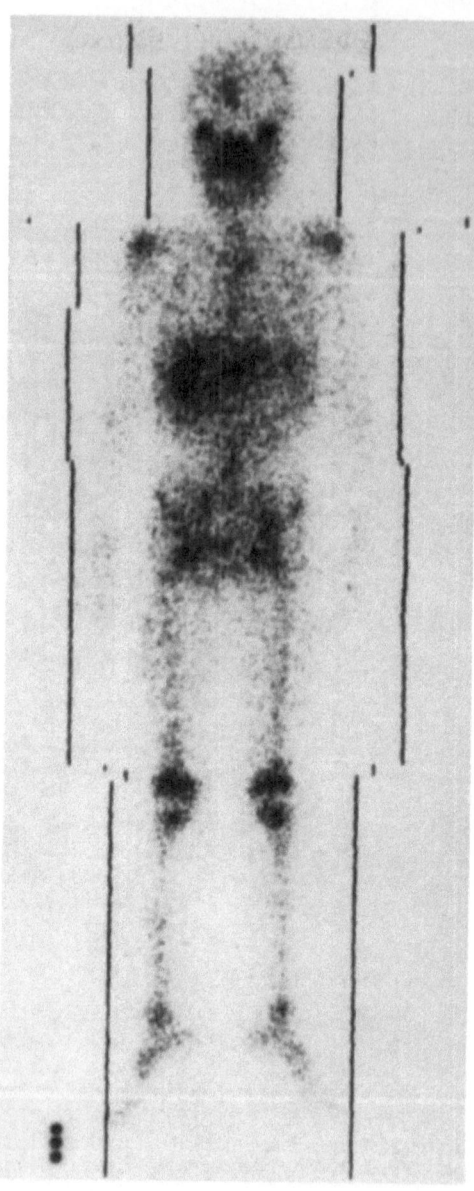

Fig. 4-3A. Anterior whole body 67-Ga scintigram of a 10-year-old girl with a Ewing's sarcoma of the right tibia. Scan shows increased 67-Ga accumulation in the right tibia corresponding to the location of the primary tumor. There is also a large area of increased nuclide uptake in the right mid-frontal area of the skull, a metastatic site of Ewing's sarcoma (See Fig. 6-9). This latter area was clinically unsuspected.

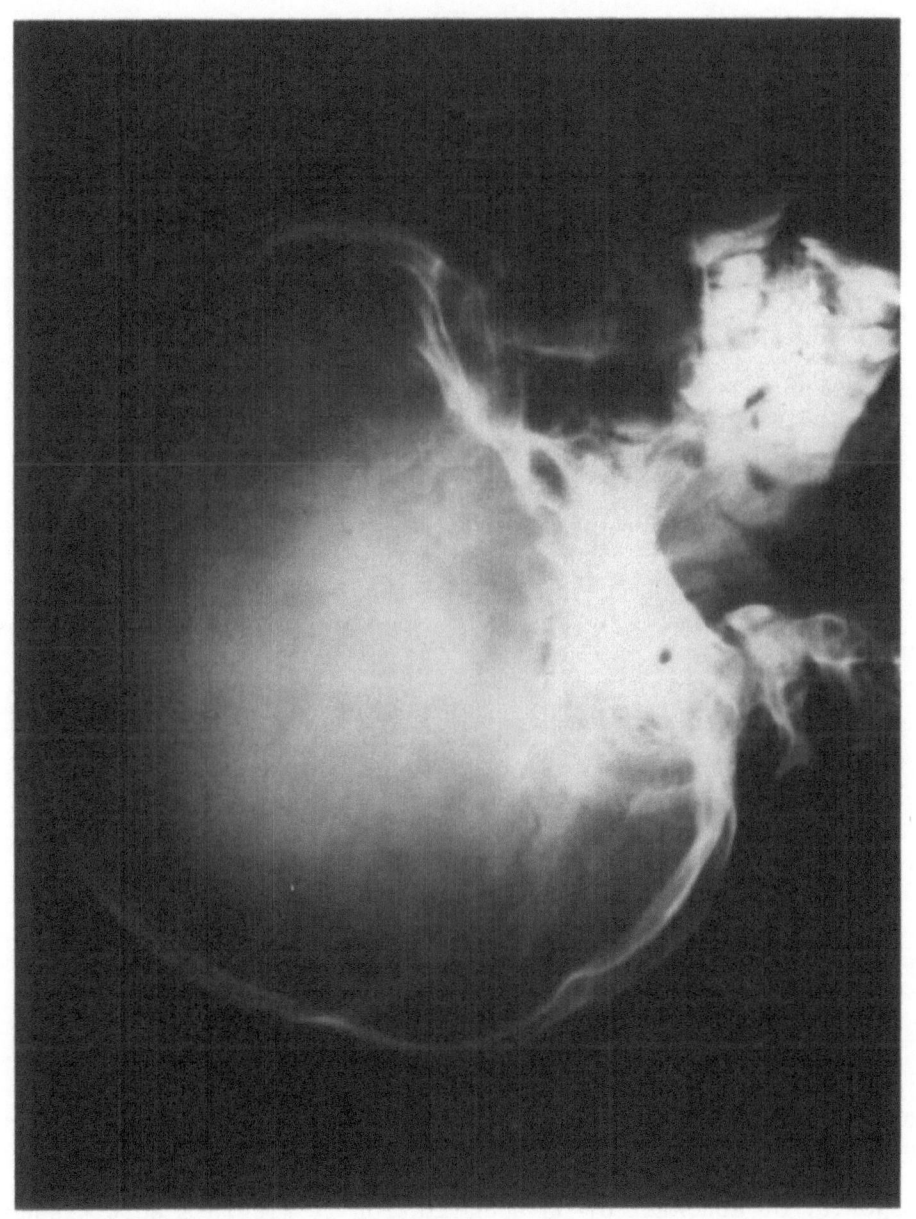

Fig. 4-3B. Ewing's sarcoma (continued): (See Fig. 4-3A.) A roentgenogram of the skull shows no abnormalities.

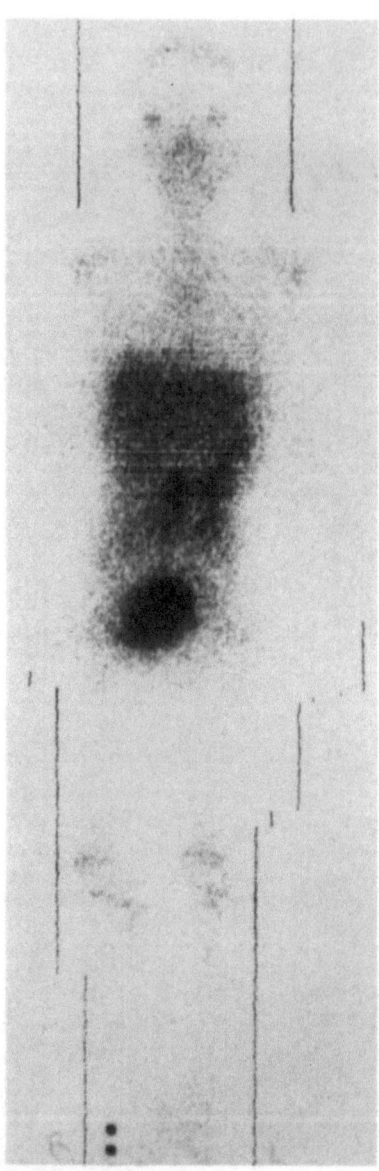

Fig. 4-4A. This patient was a 12-year-old girl with a Ewing's
sarcoma of the right ischium. The anterior whole body 67-Ga scan
shows a large accumulation of nuclide in the pelvis. Correlation
with the fluorine-18 skeletal scintigram (Fig. 4-4B) reveals that
the majority of abnormal 67-Ga accumulation is within a soft tissue
mass associated with the patient's ischial tumor. This is shown by
the elevated nuclide-filled bladder on the bone scintigram. 67-Ga
scanning in this patient revealed a greater extent of involvement
by tumor than was initially expected from the bone scan alone.

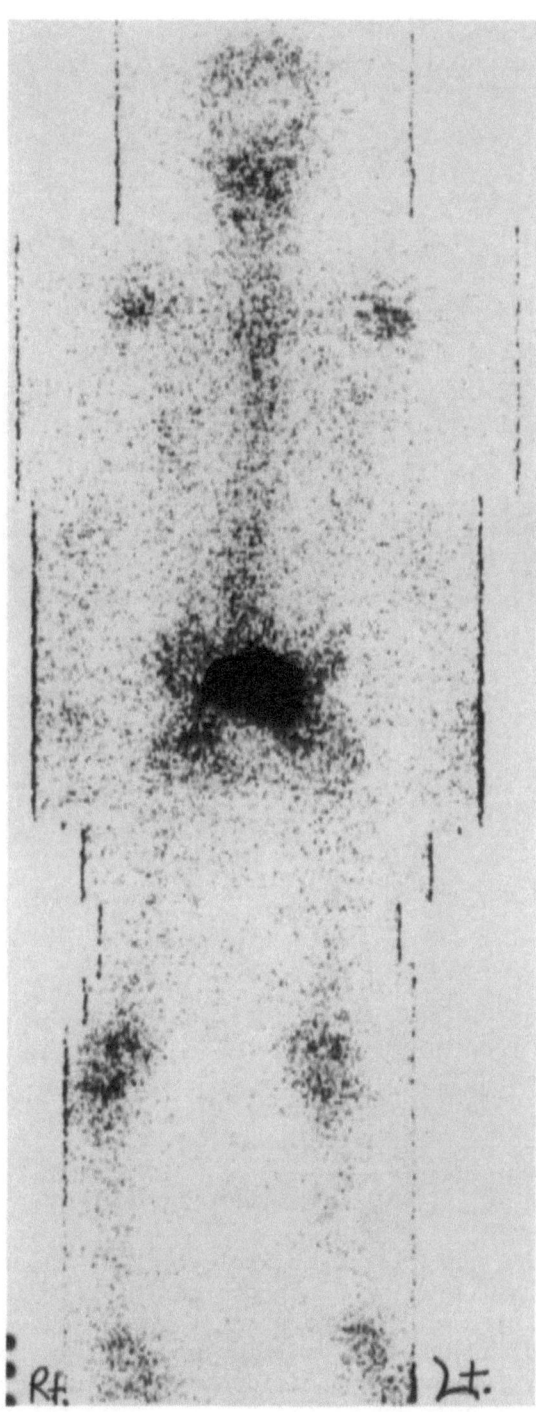

Fig. 4-4B

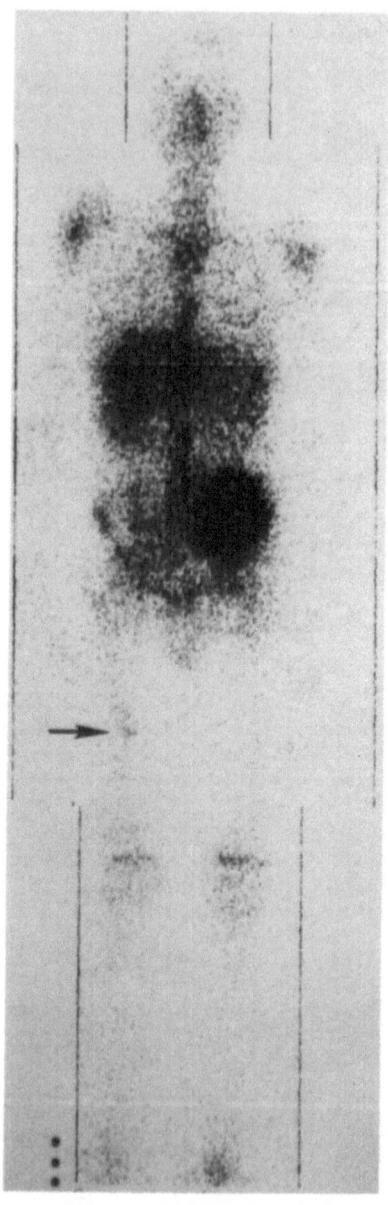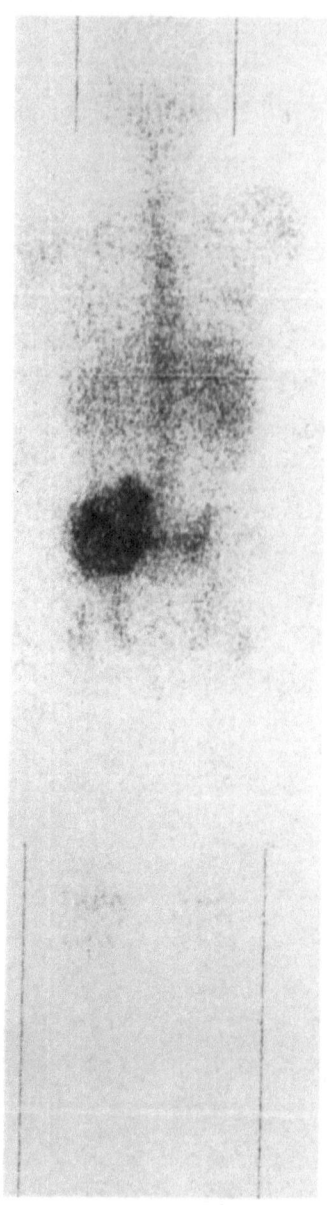

Fig. 4-5. Anterior and posterior whole body 67-Ga scintigrams of
a 19-year-old man with Ewing's sarcoma of the left ilium. The
primary tumor is seen as a large area of increased 67-Ga accumulation in the left ilium. In addition, there is a small focus of
abnormal activity (arrow) in the midshaft of the right femur. This
latter area was not seen on x-rays of the femur but was biopsied
and found to represent metastatic tumor.

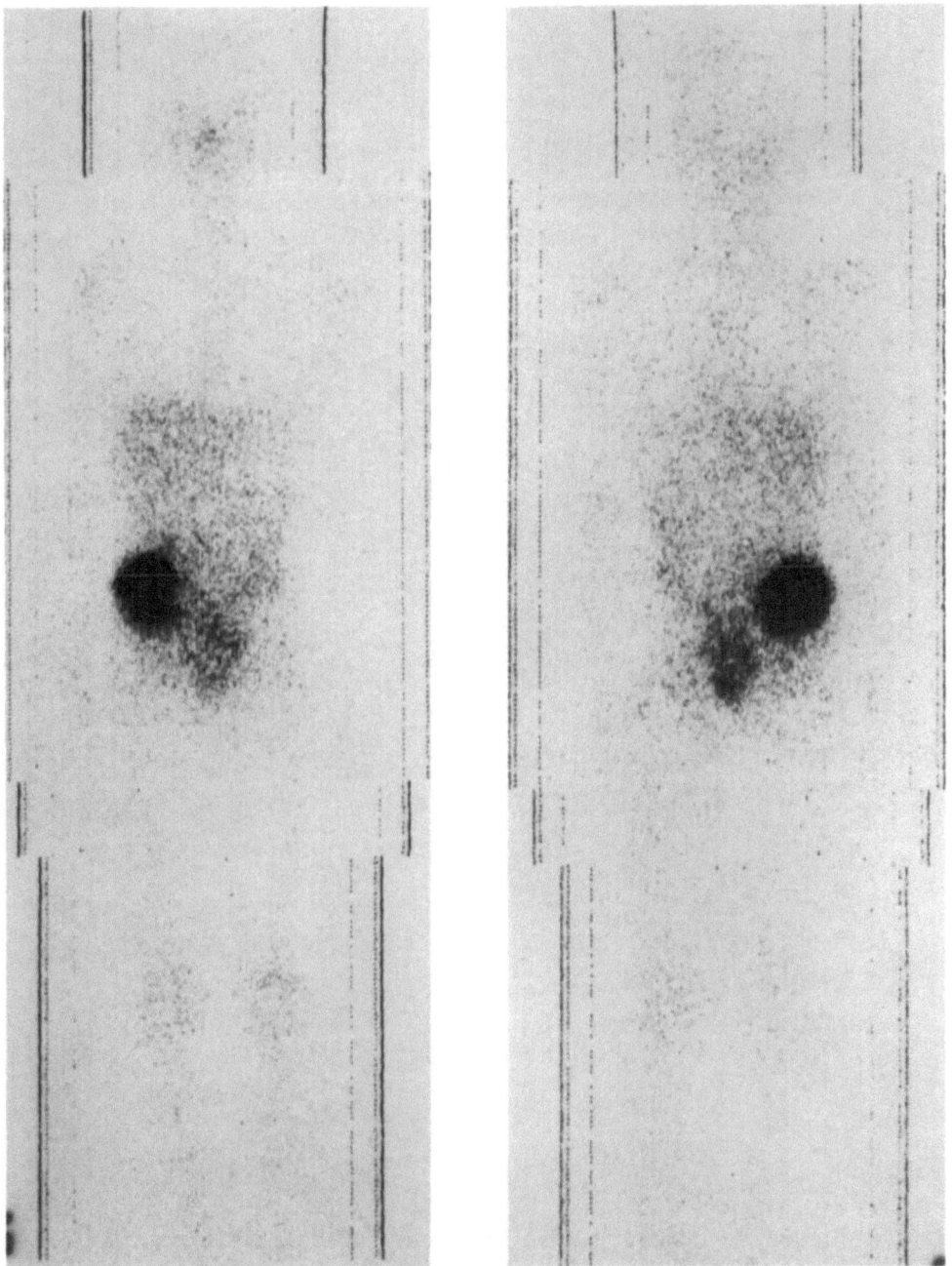

Fig. 4-6. Anterior and posterior whole body scans showing abnormal 67-Ga accumulation in the right ilium. This 16-year-old boy had a Ewing's sarcoma of the right ilium without evidence of metastases on this study.

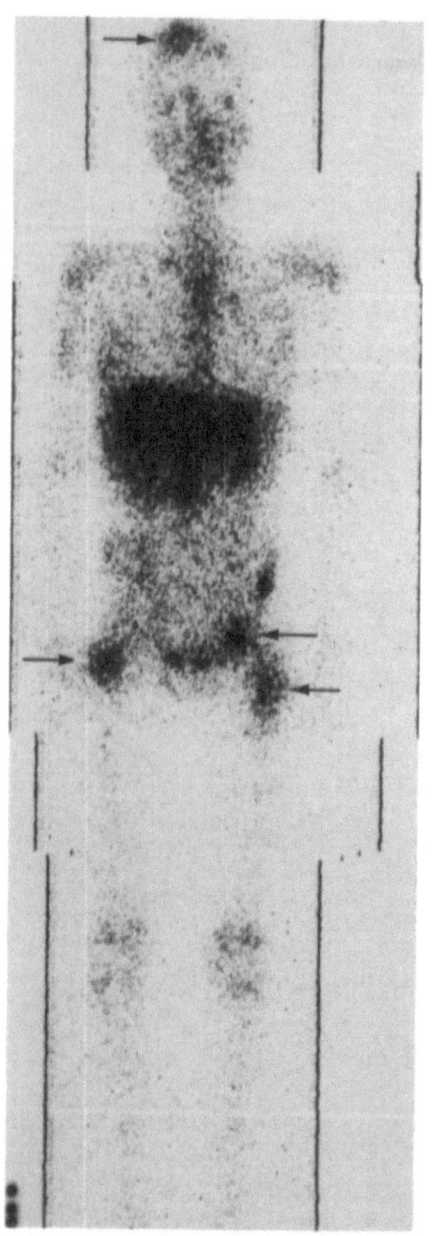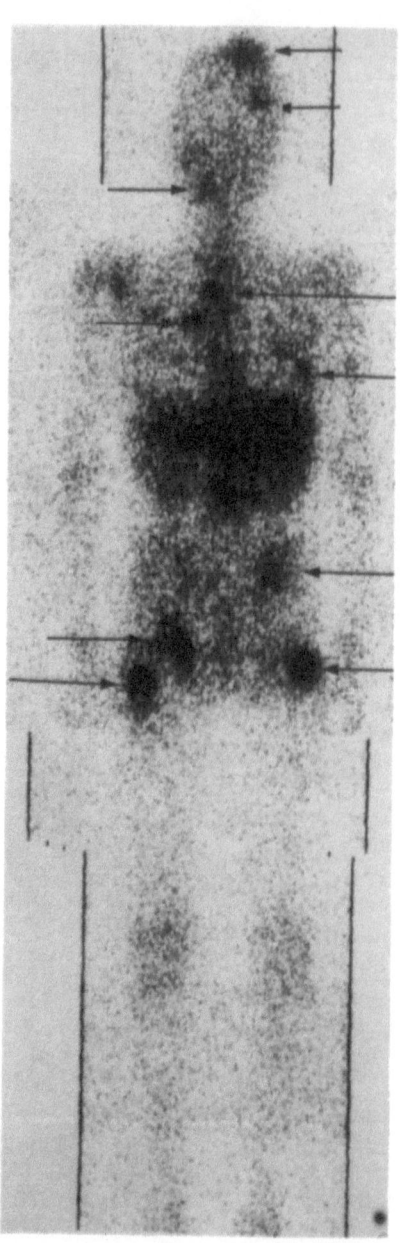

Fig. 4-7. Same patient, as in Fig. 4-6, 11 months later. Anterior
and posterior whole body views now show the following abnormal
areas of nuclide accumulation: (arrows) skull, left mandible,
mediastinum, left hilum, right and left pleura, right sacro-iliac
region, left ischium, and femoral heads bilaterally. Note on the
anterior view, there is decreased activity at the site of the
patient's primary tumor representing past irradiation effect.

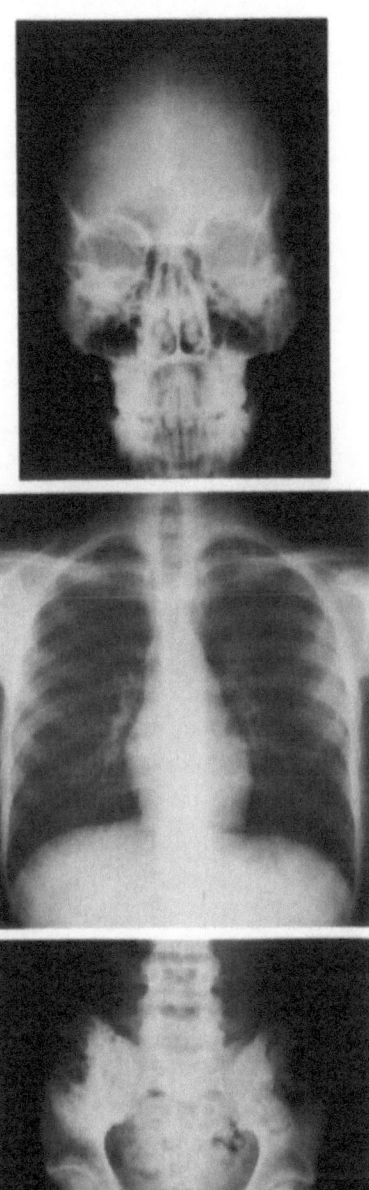

Fig. 4-8. Representative roentgenograms of this patient (Figs. 4-6 and 4-7) obtained at the same time as the 67-Ga scan in Fig. 4-7. The only detected abnormality was in the patient's primary tumor of the ilium. None of the metastases are detected.

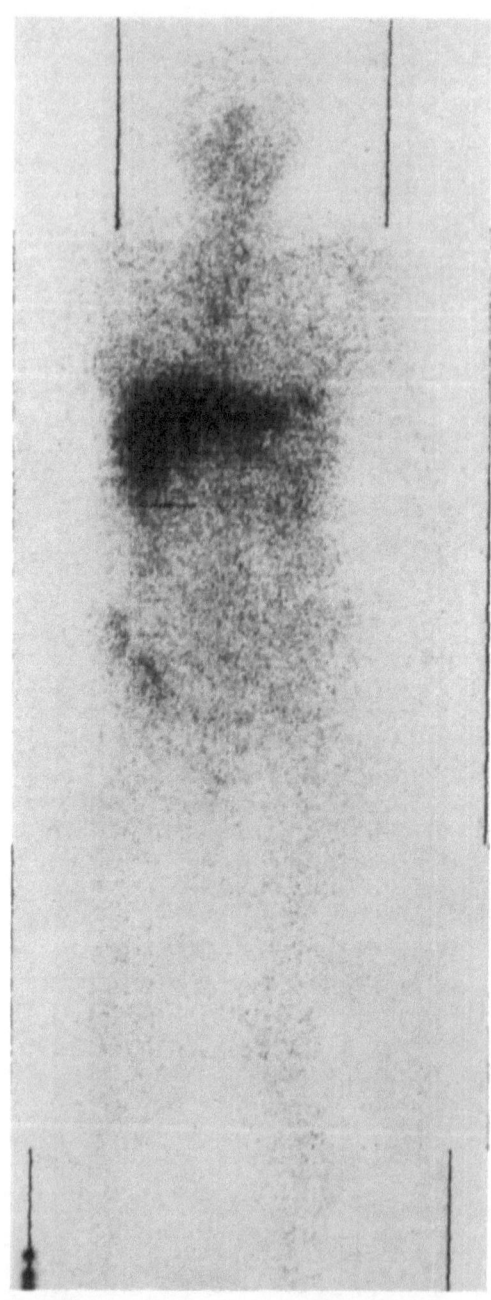

Fig. 4-9. Fifty-four-year-old woman with an osteogenic sarcoma of the right ilium thought to be secondary to remote thorotrast administration. The anterior whole body 67-Ga scan shows increased localization of nuclide in the right ilium. No metastases were detected.

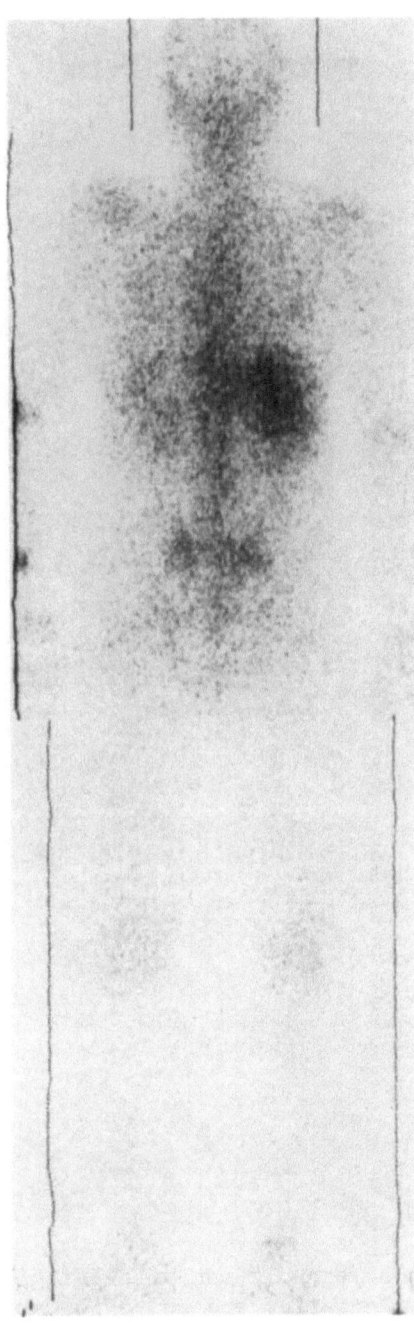

Fig. 4-10. Posterior whole body 67-Ga scan of a 19-year-old man.
There is increased localization in the distal third of the forearm
on the left. Biopsy revealed a fibrosarcoma of the left ulna.
Activity proximal to lesion is 67-Ga injection site.

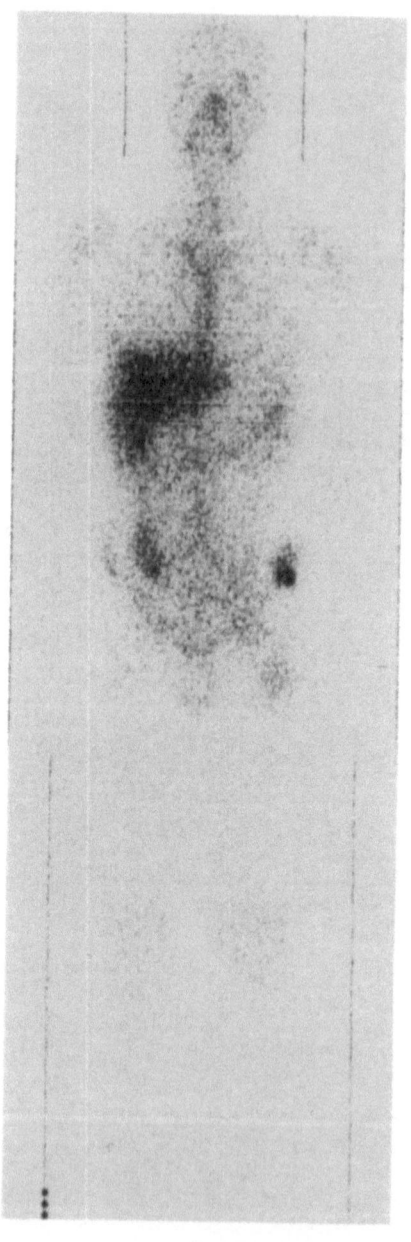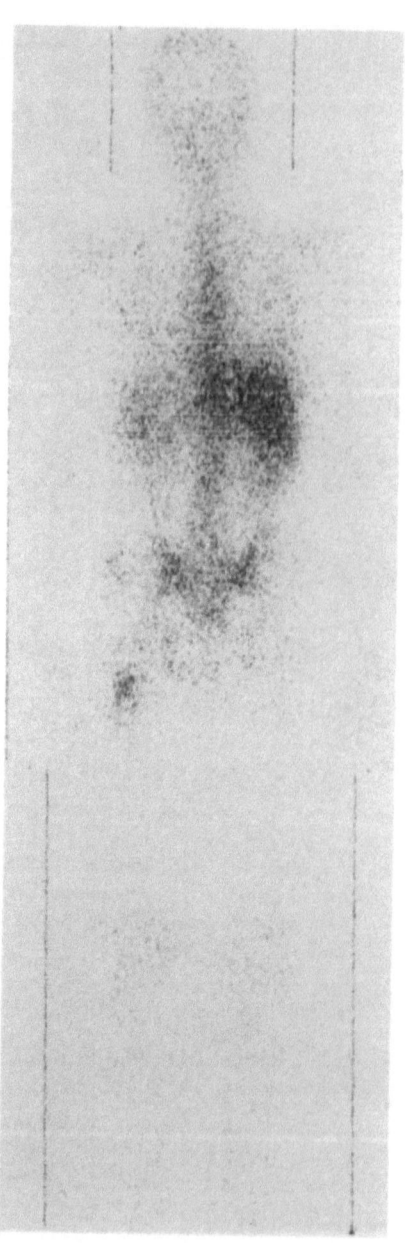

Fig. 4-11. Twenty-one-year-old man with Ewing's sarcoma of the
left proximal femur. Anterior and posterior whole body scans with
67-Ga reveal two areas of increased uptake: in the left anterior
iliac crest and in the left posterior proximal femur. The iliac
crest activity is secondary to a previous excision of bone from
that area for use as a bone pack. The proximal femur activity is
in the patient's primary tumor.

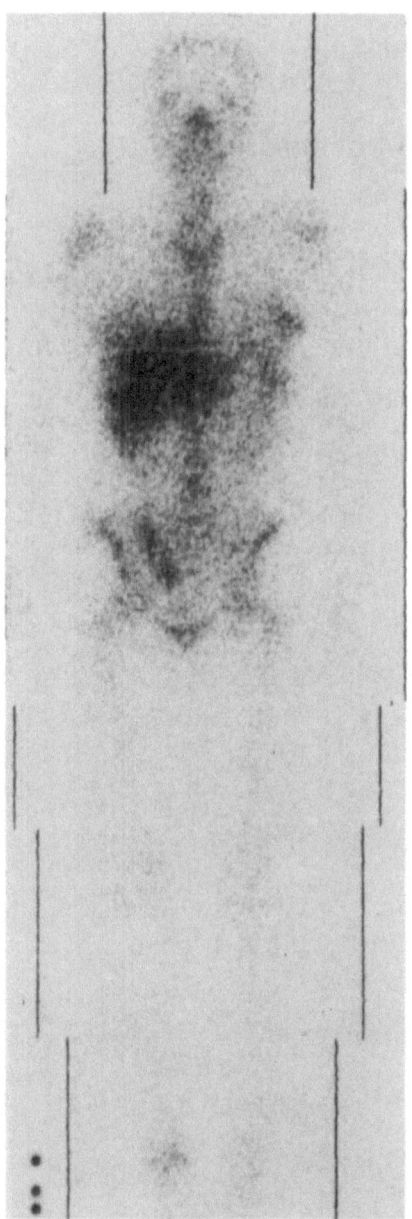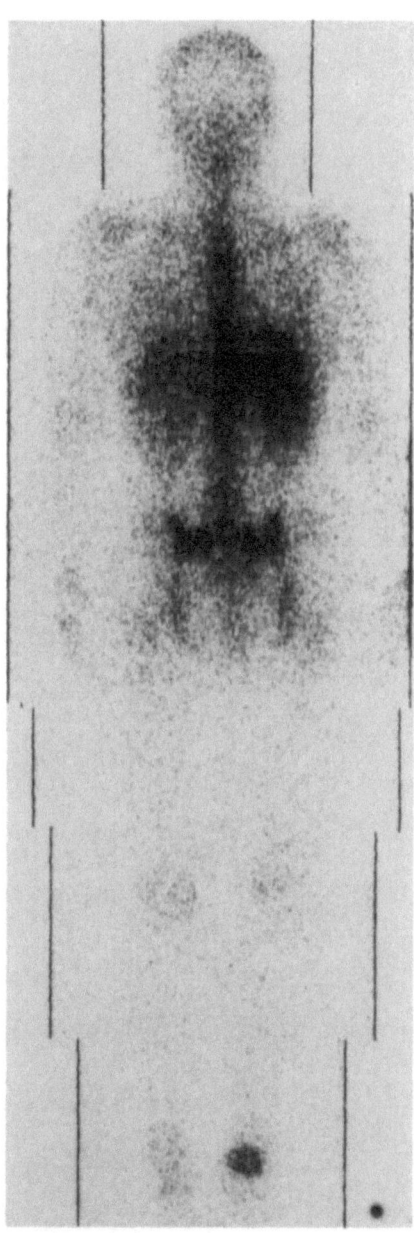

Fig. 4-12. Anterior and posterior whole body 67-Ga scintigrams of a 19-year-old woman with Ewing's sarcoma of the right os calcis. The increased nuclide uptake in the region of the right ankle represents the patient's primary tumor. There is also a band-like area of increased 67-Ga activity in the right lower quadrant of the abdomen which remained after serial post-laxative views and was therefore thought to represent an abnormal accumulation.

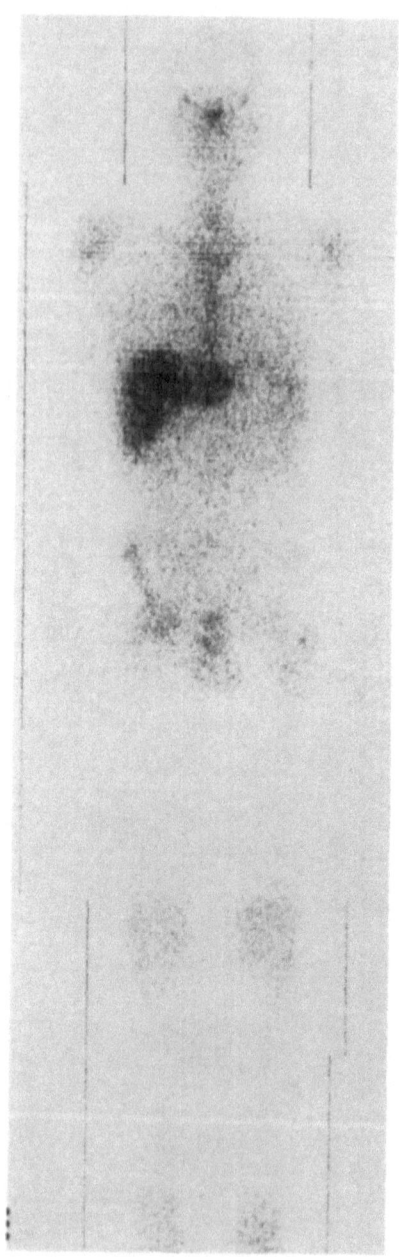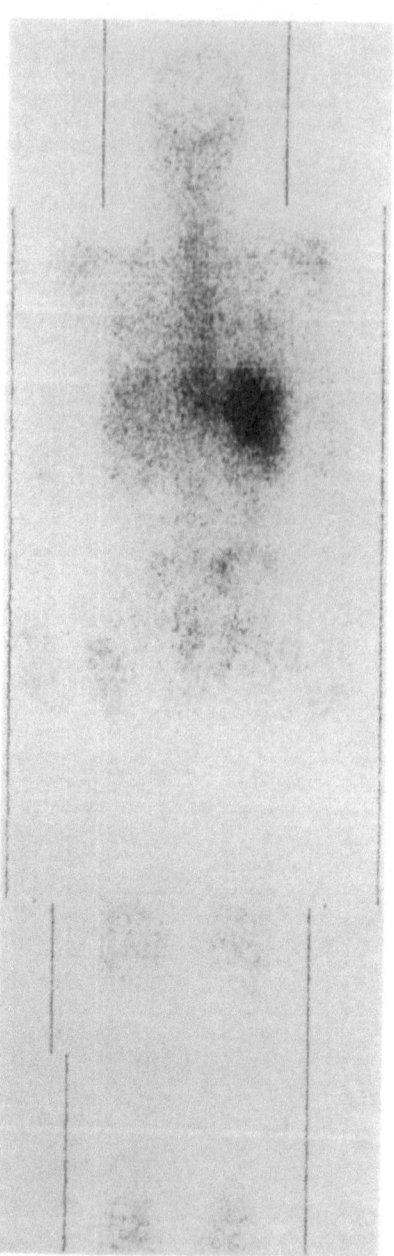

Fig. 4-13. Sixteen-year-old boy with a previously radiated Ewing's sarcoma of the left ilium. Follow-up anterior and posterior whole body 67-Ga scintigrams show decreased uptake in the region of the radiated left ilium anteriorly and left sacrum posteriorly. Decreased 67-Ga uptake is a frequent finding following radiation therapy.

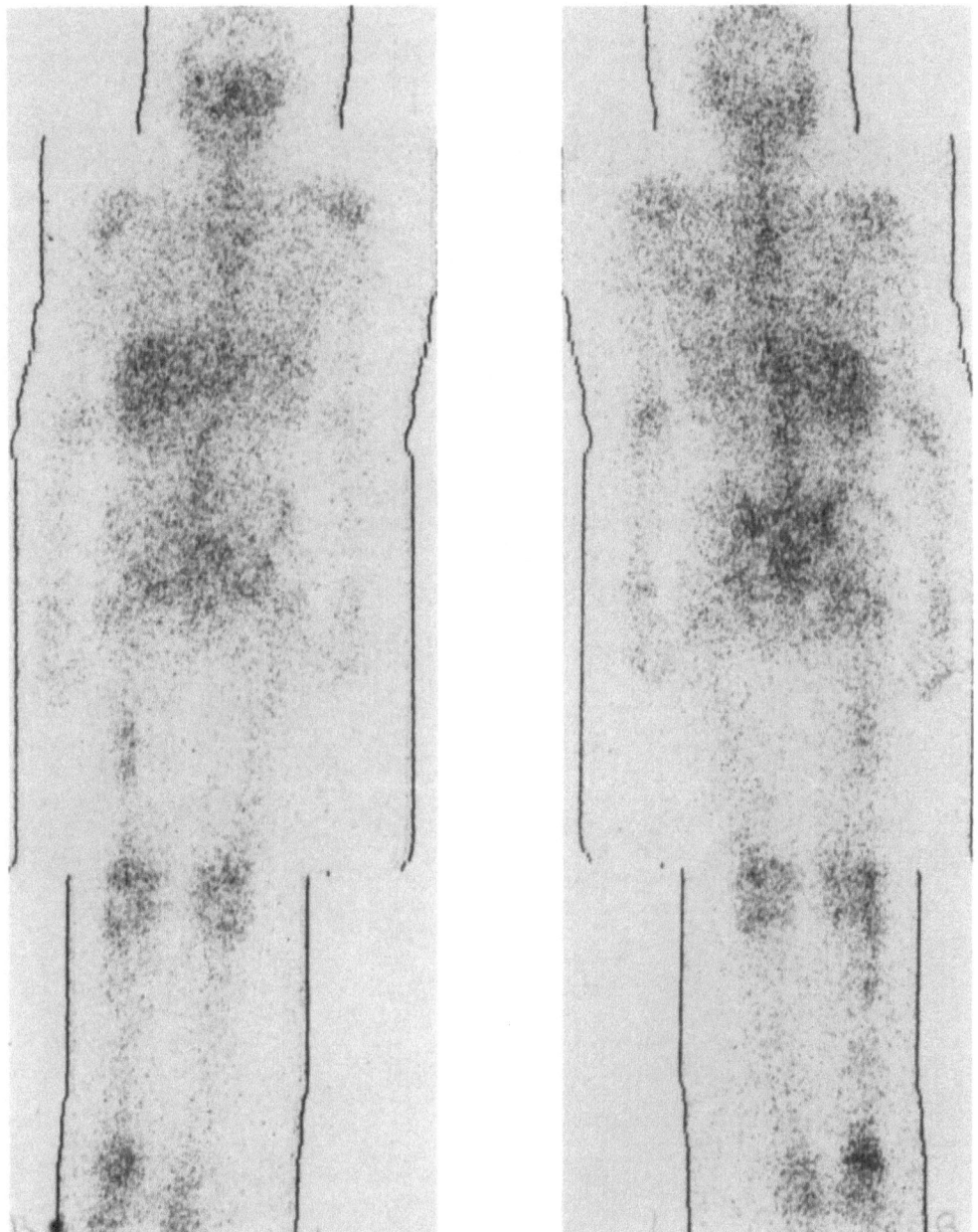

Fig. 4-14. Anterior and posterior whole body 67-Ga scans of a
16-year-old boy with suspected Ewing's sarcoma of the right tibia
and fibula. Scans show increased uptake in the region of the
tibia and fibula as well as in the shaft of the right mid-femur.
This latter area was later proved to contain tumor although it was
unsuspected both clinically and radiologically.

CHAPTER 5

Lung Tumors

Robert J. Kramer, M. D.

Department of Nuclear Medicine, Clinical Center

National Institutes of Health, Bethesda, Maryland

Research on the tumor-localizing radioisotope 67-Ga citrate reveals both bone and soft-tissue-seeking properties. Bone localization is apparent by the ability of the nuclide to demonstrate the majority of primary bone tumors. The soft-tissue affinity of this isotope can be illustrated by its uptake in pulmonary neoplasms which represent one of the most consistently visualized soft-tissue tumors. The data reported by Hayes (13) indicate a 68% rate of positive scans in all tumor types studied, with lung and lymphoma subgroups having better results. A recent literature review showed that 194 of 228 (85%) documented cases of lung neoplasms were positive on 67-Ga scanning (1). There is, however, no apparent difference in 67-Ga uptake by lung tumors of various histologic types (24,66).

A major contribution of 67-Ga scanning in pulmonary malignancies lies in the performance of sequential studies. The assumption of this technique is that only viable neoplastic tissue can concentrate 67-Ga. Hayes and Edwards demonstrated necrotic neoplastic tissue had less 67-Ga accumulation than viable tumors. Higasi has also shown an inverse relationship of 67-Ga tumor uptake and radiation dose (20). The occurrence of a negative 67-Ga scintigram following treatment of a tumor is therefore presently considered to indicate adequate treatment, while a continued positive study implies recurrent disease or inadequate therapy.

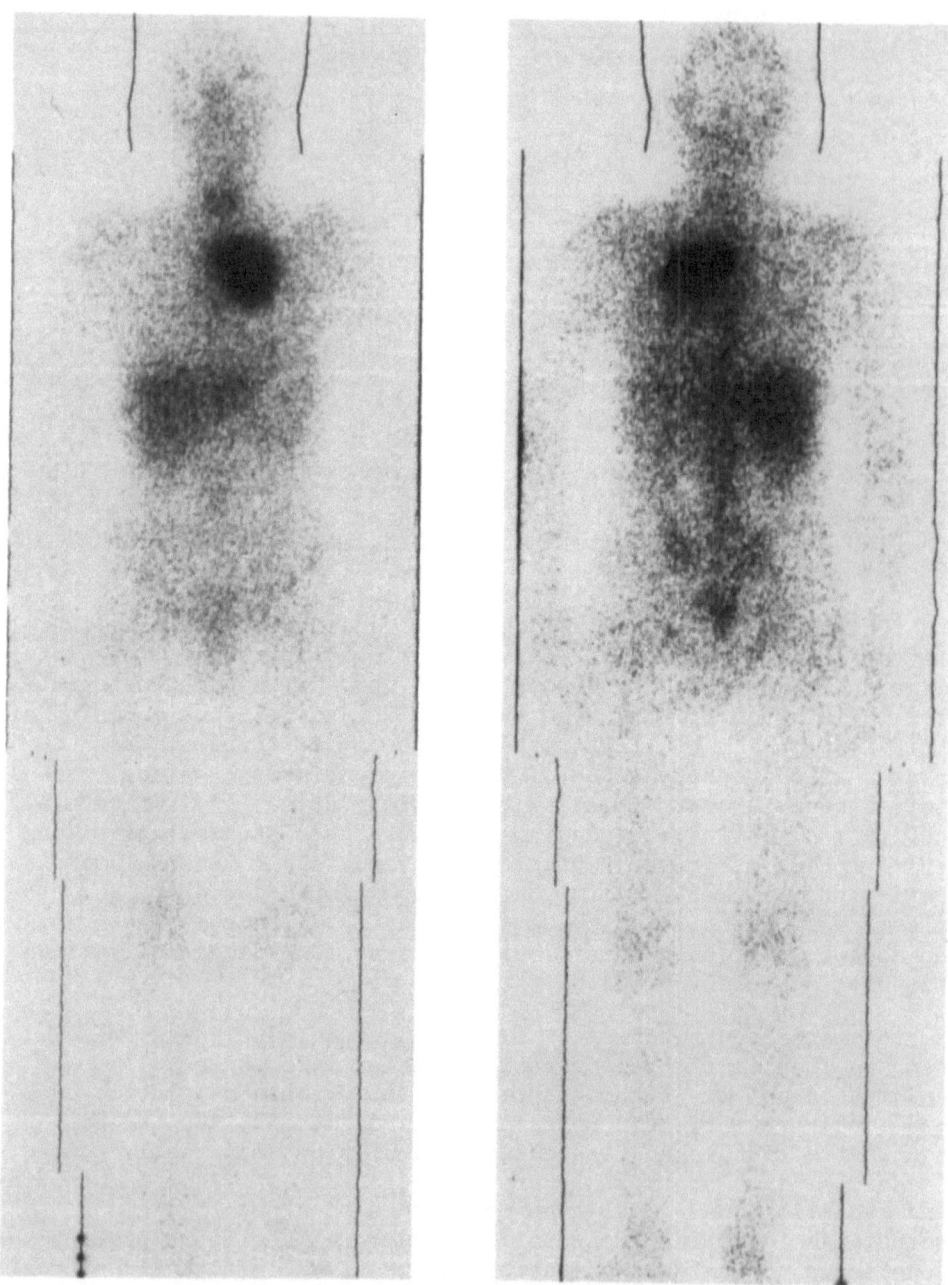

Fig. 5-1. Anterior and posterior whole body 67-Ga scans of a
48-year-old white male with a carcinoma of the lung. The 67-Ga
study reveals dense nuclide accumulation in a large right hilar
mass. This central tumor localization is typical of squamous
cell carcinoma.

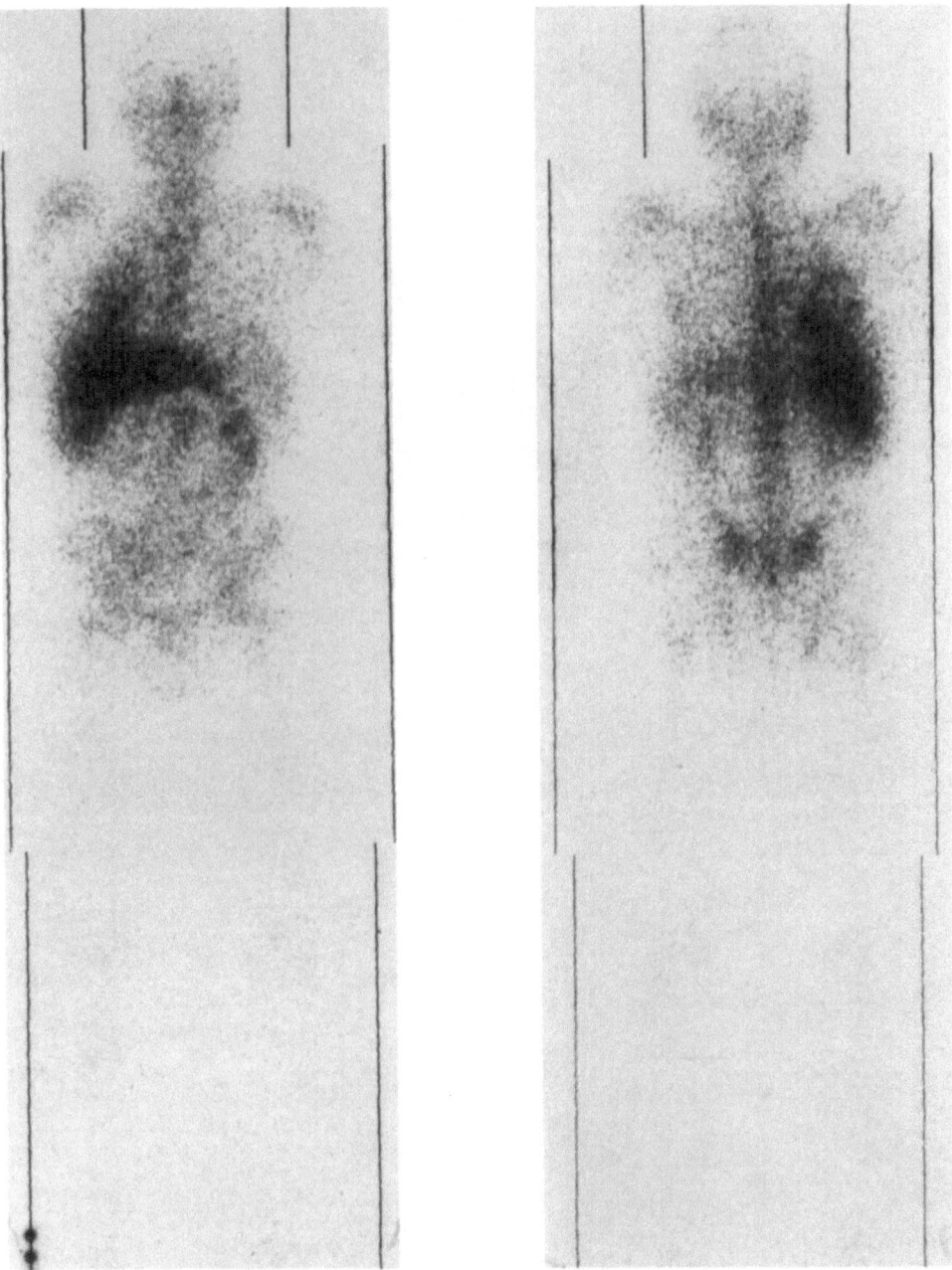

Fig. 5-2. 67-Ga photoscans of a 42-year-old white male with carcinoma of the lung. Both anterior and posterior views demonstrate 67-Ga uptake in right lower lung field adjacent to the diaphragm. This peripheral tumor localization is typical of adenocarcinoma.

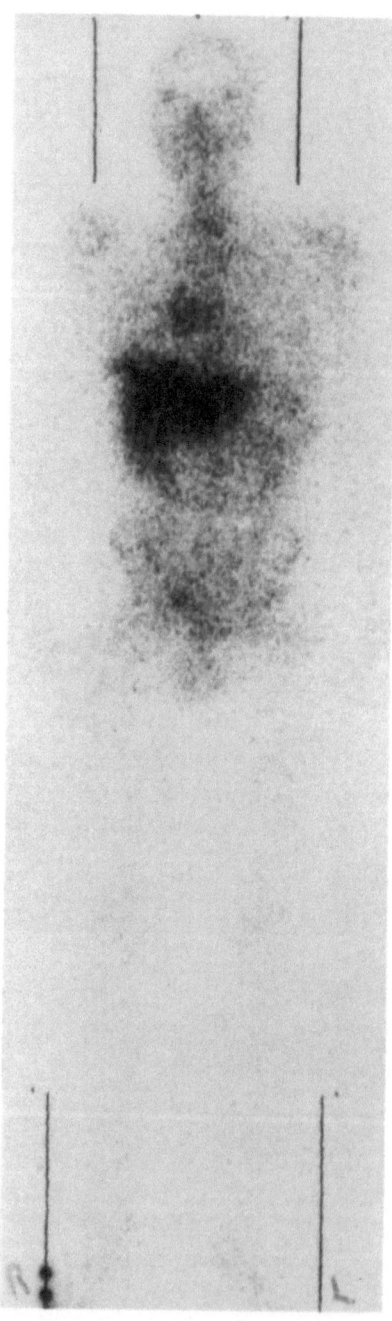

Fig. 5-3A. Lung Carcinoma: Sequential Studies.
Thirty-eight-year-old white male with bronchogenic carcinoma
treated with radiotherapy. This initial 67-Ga scan revealed an
area of isotope accumulation in the right hilar region.

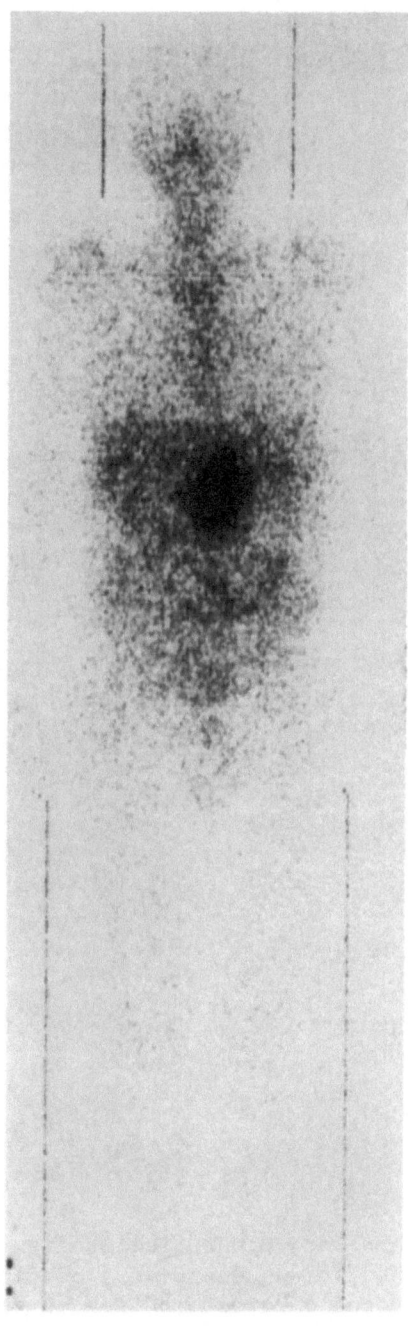

Fig. 5-3B. Three months following treatment, a repeat 67-Ga study demonstrated virtually no abnormal uptake in the thorax. There is, however, 67-Ga localization in a large epigastric mass. Lymphangiography and biopsy confirmed the presence of metastatic disease.

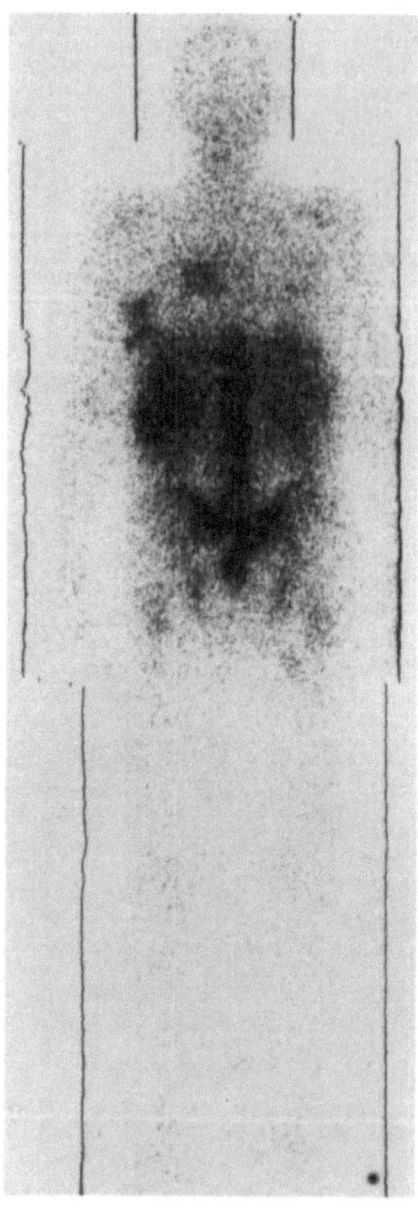

Fig. 5-4A. Lung Carcinoma: Sequential Studies.
Two posterior whole body 67-Ga scans were obtained in a 50-year-old
patient with a bronchogenic carcinoma treated surgically and with
radiotherapy. The initial study reveals residual tumor uptake of
67-Ga citrate in the left hilum. The thoracotomy site is also
visualized. The absence of tracer uptake in the thoracic spine
above the level of the diaphragm is most likely due to previous
radiation therapy.

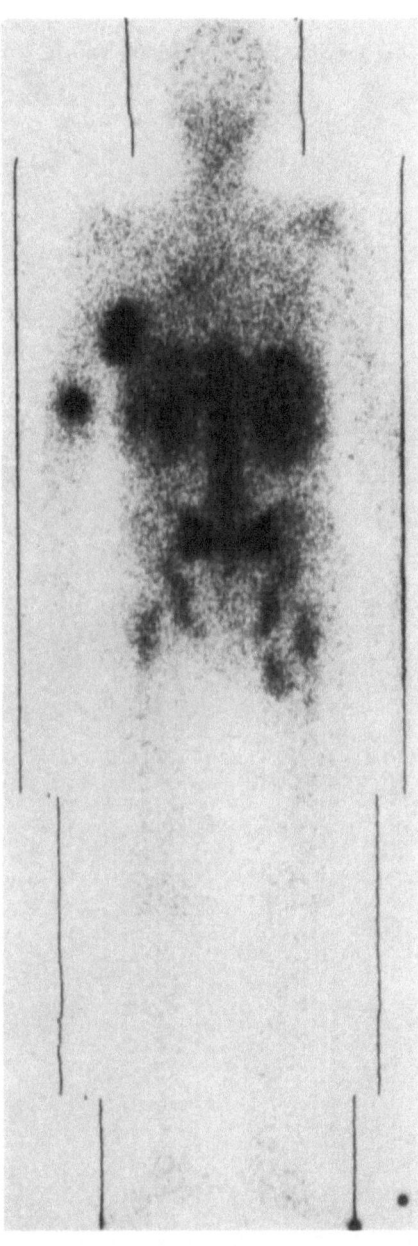

Fig. 5-4B. One month later, a repeat posterior scan reveals
further diminution of the primary hilar mass. The thoracotomy
site is still evident as well as the area of isotope administration
in the left antecubital fossa. New regions of abnormal 67-Ga
accumulation are seen in the right shoulder, right ischial area
and the soft tissues of the right upper thigh. These findings are
consistent with the presence of metastatic disease.

CHAPTER 6

Tumors of Head and Neck

Alfred E. Jones, M. D. and Gerald S. Johnston, M. D.

Department of Nuclear Medicine, Clinical Center

National Institutes of Health, Bethesda, Maryland

Experience in the use of 67-Ga for tumors of the head and neck has been limited at NIH; however, an increasing number of patients with tumors in this region are being studied. The use of 67-Ga scintigraphy for the detection of metastases from these tumors appears encouraging.

A variety of tumors of the head and neck have been evaluated with 67-Ga. Although most of the primary tumors have localized 67-Ga, it must be recognized that the primary tumor seen in these cases was often large; therefore, the object of performing 67-Ga scintigraphy was to detect regional and/or distant metastases.

Whole body rectilinear scintigraphy with 1:5 image minification was used during the early phases of the 67-Ga evaluation of patients who were known to have malignancy. Although the primary tumors were often visualized using this technique, regional metastases were rarely found and it was unusual to find distant metastases. It has proven more useful to employ the gamma camera technique, as described in Chapter 11. The gamma camera has facilitated the collection of multiple regional views and has rendered a better evaluation of metastases in regional nodes. The gamma camera technique has also been especially useful in the detection of metastatic lesions in the skull. Furthermore, 99m-Tc polyphosphate scintigraphy of the head and neck has proven helpful when 67-Ga results have been borderline.

The following scintigraphs demonstrate a variety of primary and metastatic lesions detected either by rectilinear scintigraphy (1:5 minification) or by gamma camera.

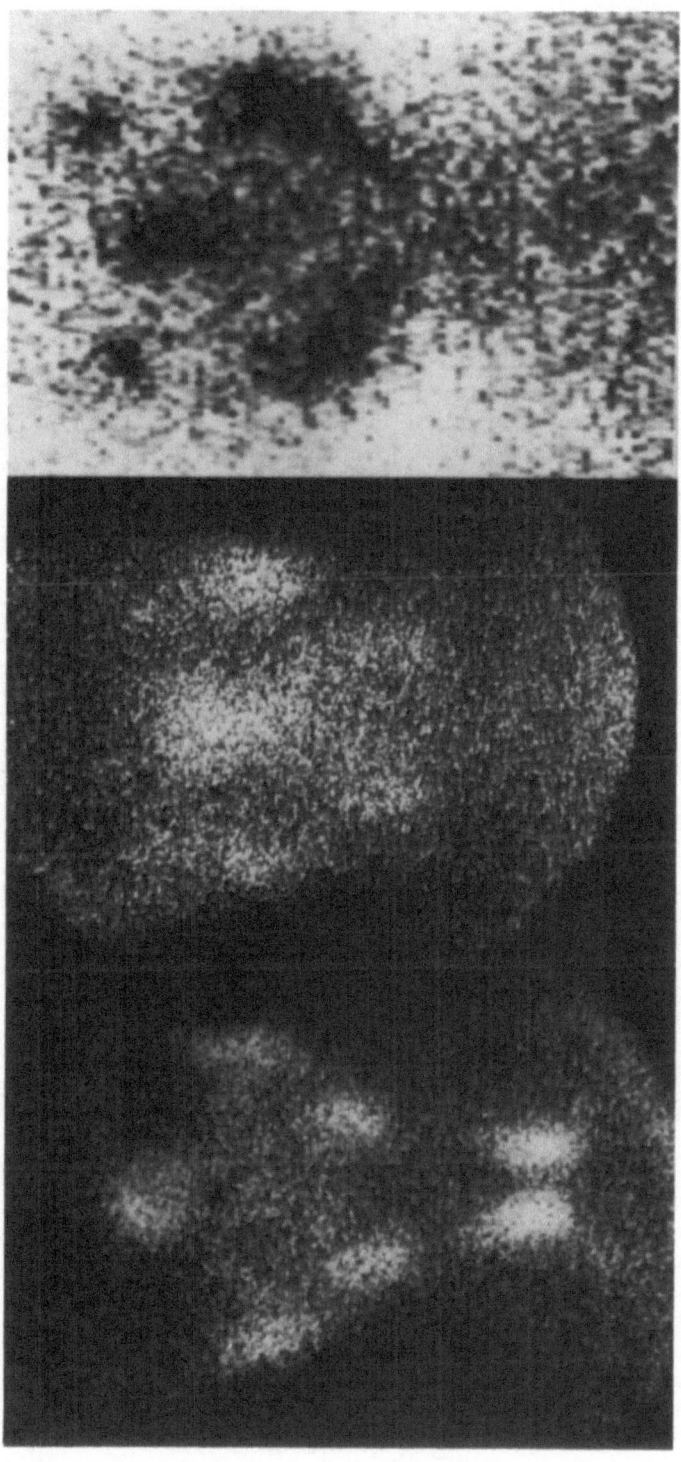

Fig. 6-1. Normal anterior scintigraphic views of head and neck: 99m-Tc pertechnetate gamma camera view (left) demonstrates the following bilaterally symmetrical structures from below upwards: lobes of the thyroid gland; submandibular salivary glands; parotid glands and centrally, the region of the nose. 67-Ga gamma camera and rectilinear views (middle and right) reveal the same structures except the thyroid gland is not seen but the lacrimal glands may be seen to a varying degree from time to time in various subjects. Refer to description accompanying Fig. 3-1.

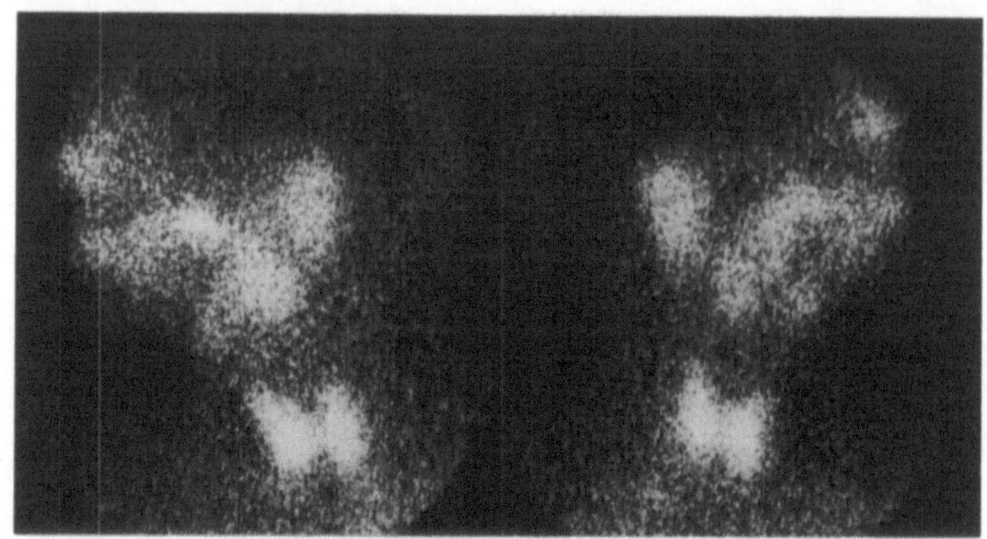

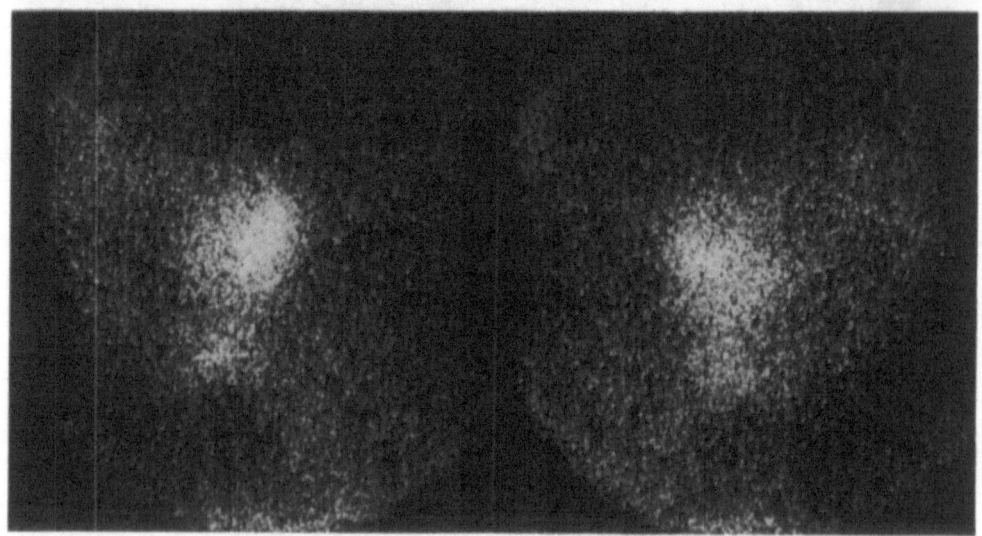

Fig. 6-2. Normal lateral gamma camera scintigrams of head and neck:
99m-Tc pertechnetate views (above) show both lobes of the thyroid
gland and directly above, the submandibular glands, and above that,
the parotid glands are seen. Activity is also seen within the mouth
and the tip of the nose. 67-Ga scintigrams (below) show only the
submandibular and parotid glands. The lacrimal gland is faintly
seen in this instance. The lateral portion of the neck, seen below
the submandibular gland, may reveal 67-Ga localized in cervical
nodes when they are involved with tumor (Fig. 6-4).

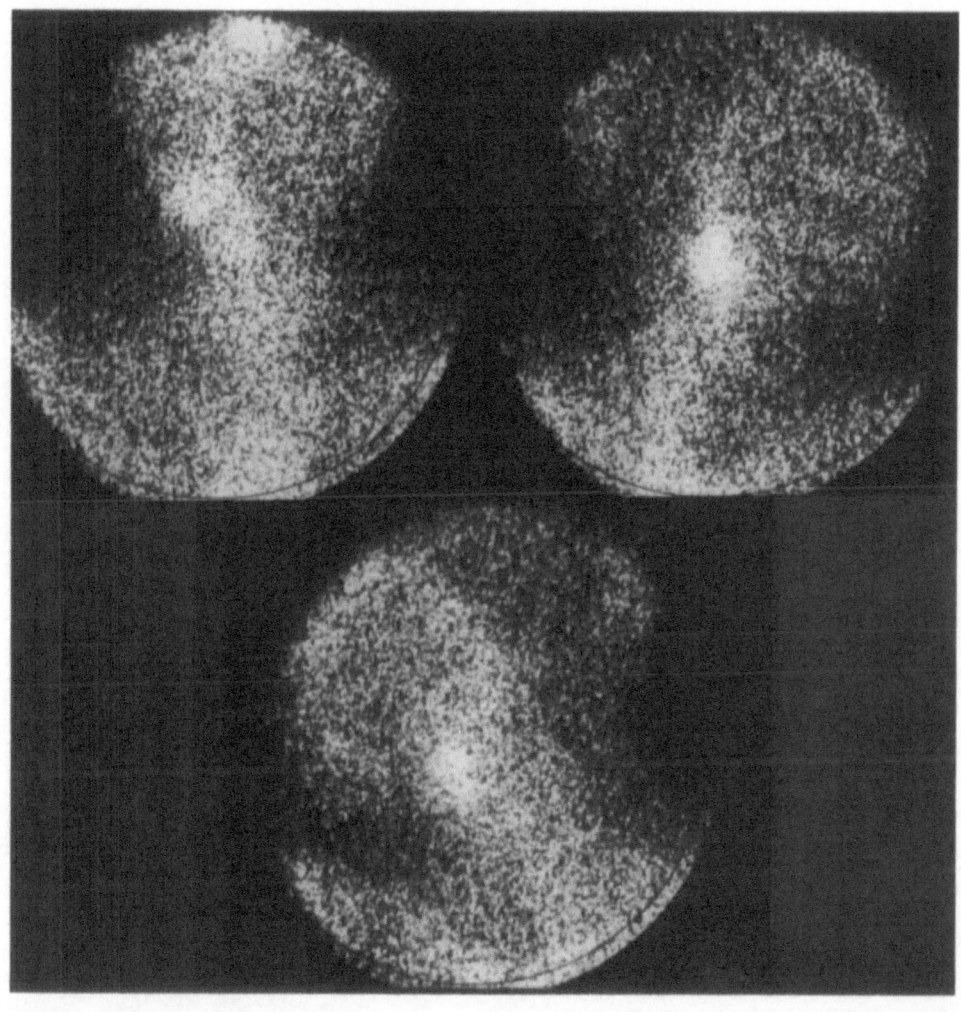

Fig. 6-3. Fifty-year-old man with carcinoma of the larynx and palpable right neck nodes: 67-Ga scintigrams include anterior and right lateral (above); left lateral (below). Note that there is an area of 67-Ga localization in the right side of the jaw and right neck on the anterior view (above left). This same region is also seen on both lateral views but more prominently on the right. 67-Ga localization in the neck may represent lymph node involvement (See Fig. 6-4).

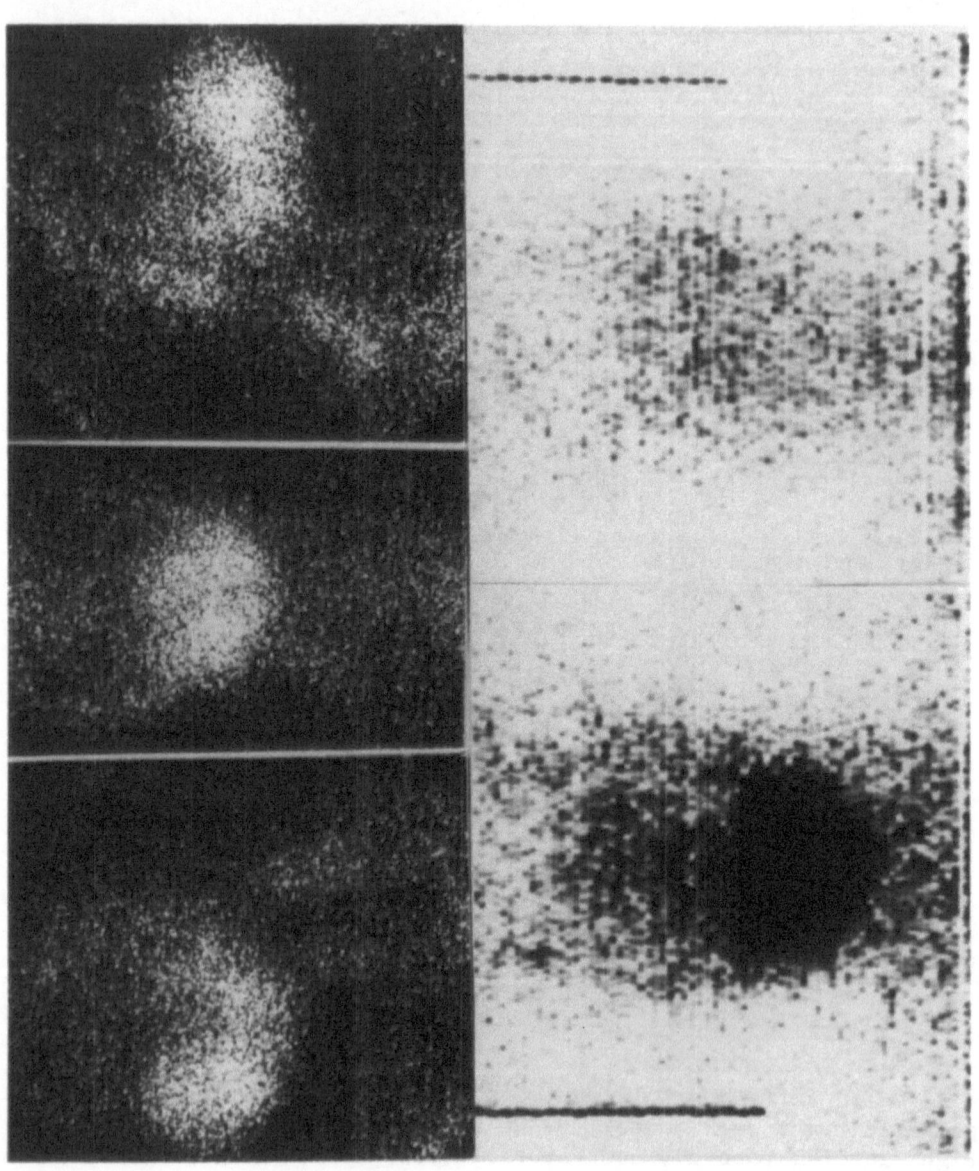

Fig. 6-4. 16-year-old girl with high floor of mouth tumor: There is extension into the anterior jaw with bilateral neck nodes. Upper three scintigrams were obtained with a gamma camera. The lower two are dual probe anterior and posterior rectilinear scintigrams of the same patient. The neck nodes are especially prominent in the right lateral view but are not evident in the rectilinear views. Gamma camera scintigrams have proved helpful when tumor is known or suspected in the head or neck.

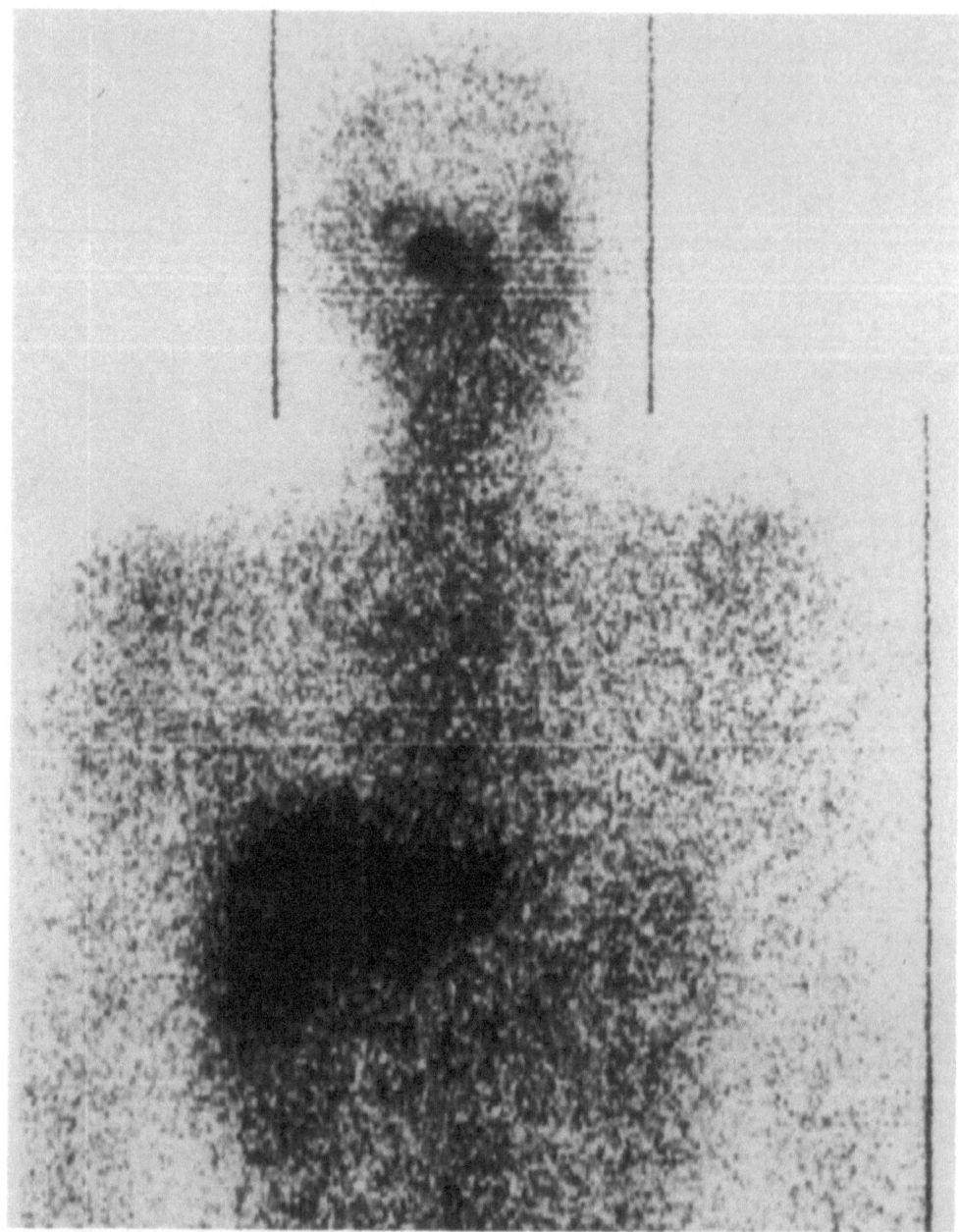

Fig. 6-5. 38-year-old man with adenocarcinoma of the right parotid
gland excised with right radical neck dissection eight years prior
to the above 67-Ga anterior rectilinear scan. This image demonstrates the recurrence of tumor below the right eye. While there
is no discrete localization of 67-Ga in the neck there is a generalized increase of activity on the entire right side of the neck.

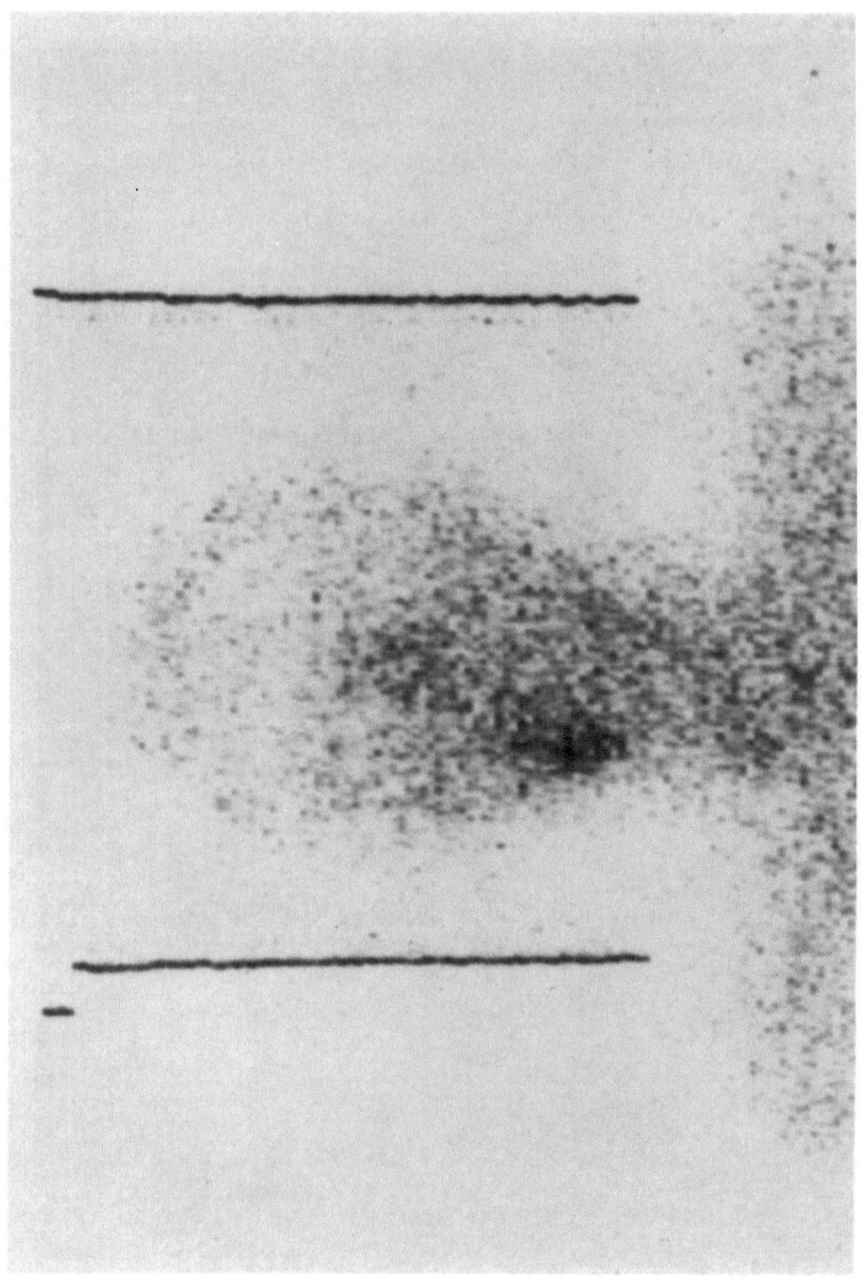

Fig. 6-6. Carcinoma of the floor of the mouth in a 57-year-old man. This anterior rectilinear scintigram has detected the primary tumor. There is no increase in activity on either side of the neck in contrast to Fig. 6-5.

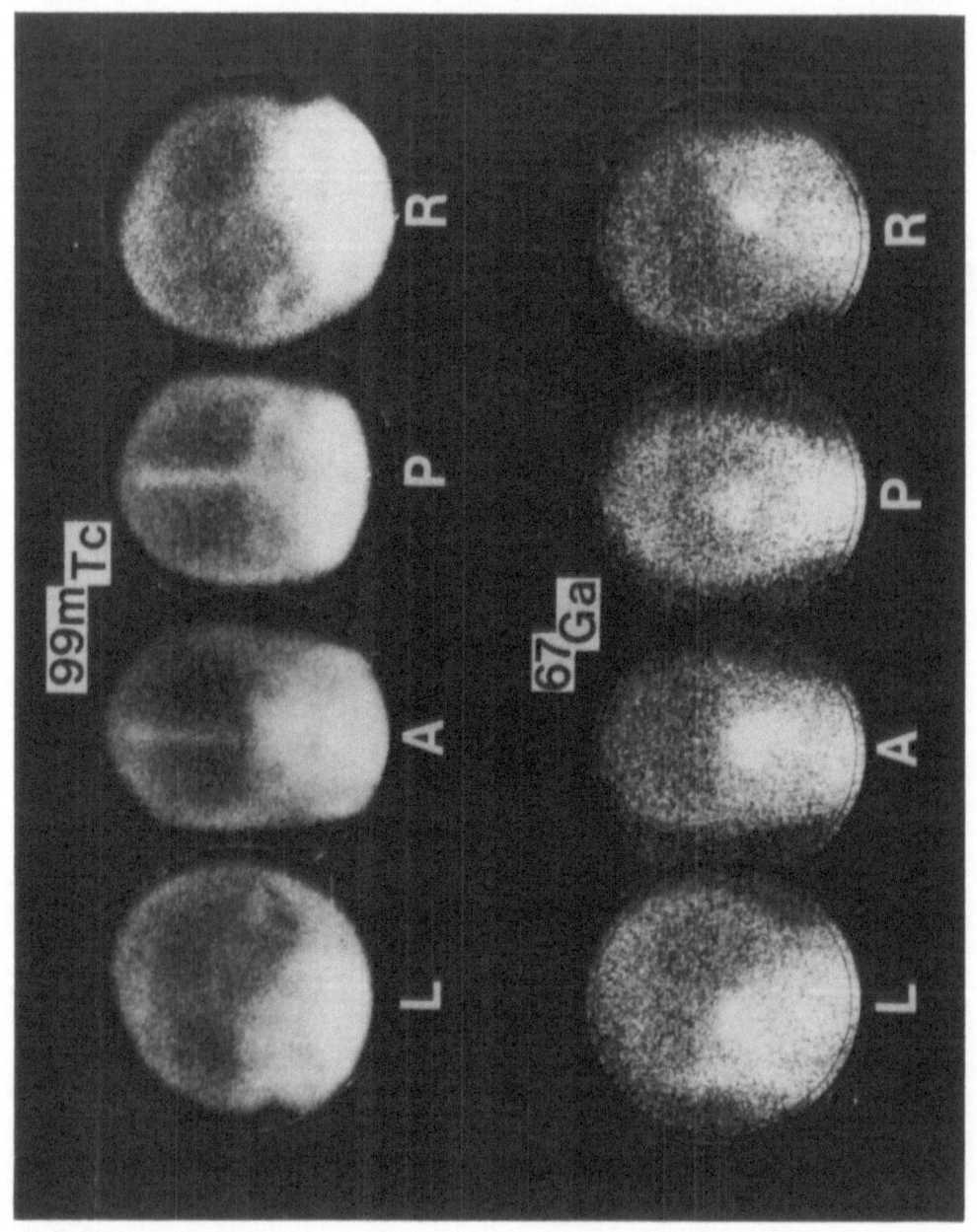

Fig. 6-7. Comparative 99m-Tc pertechnetate and 67-Ga scintigrams in a 42-year-old woman with adenocystic carcinoma of the sphenoid sinus. The 99m-Tc pertechnetate study was interpreted as normal; however, the 67-Ga views show tumor localization in both lateral views. The tumor is close to midline and can be mistaken for normal nasopharyngeal localization of 67-Ga on the anterior view. The posterior view with 99m-Tc pertechnetate indicates activity in the posterior fossa below the lateral sinuses. This is sometimes seen normally and may be attributed to oropharyngeal activity related to high salivary levels of 99m-Tc pertechnetate being secreted into the oral cavity. It could also represent the tumor. The 67-Ga study clarified this interpretive dilemma. L = left; A = anterior; P = posterior; R = right.

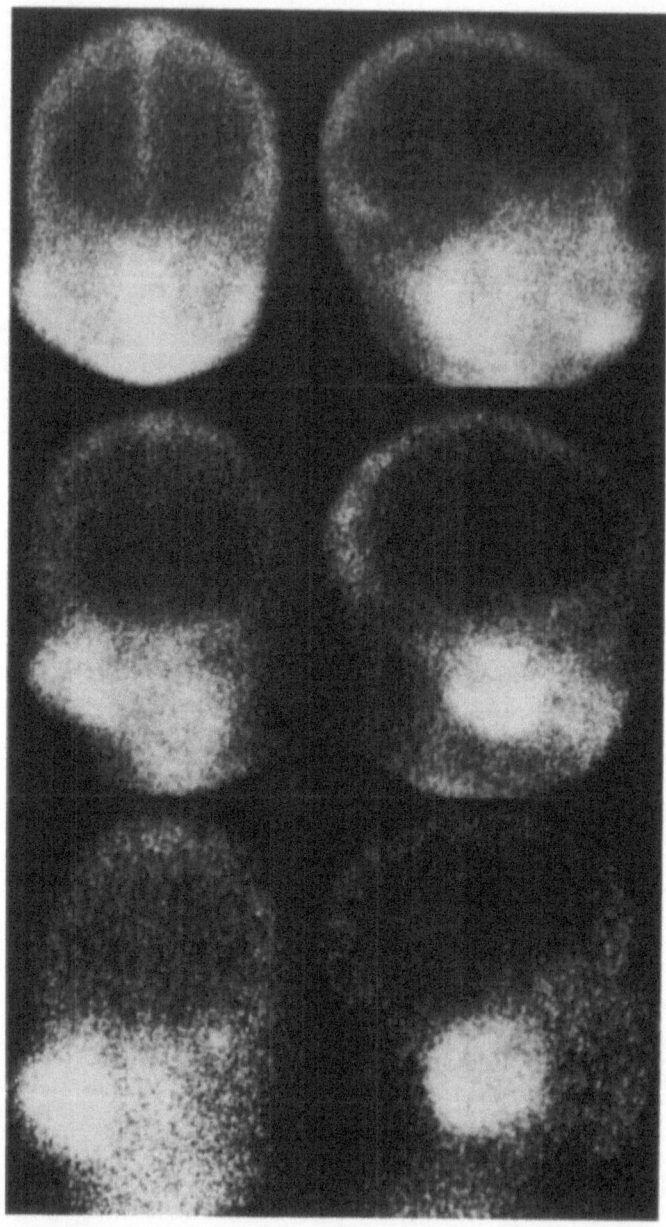

Fig. 6-8. Right preauricular swelling in a 21-year-old man found to have a chondrosarcoma of the right mandible. All three radio-pharmaceuticals revealed the lesion; 99m-Tc pertechnetate (above), 99m-Tc polyphosphate (middle), and 67-Ga (below). The tumor which is clearly seen with 67-Ga has a bony component and is therefore prominently demonstrated by 99m-Tc polyphosphate. Compare with Fig. 6-9.

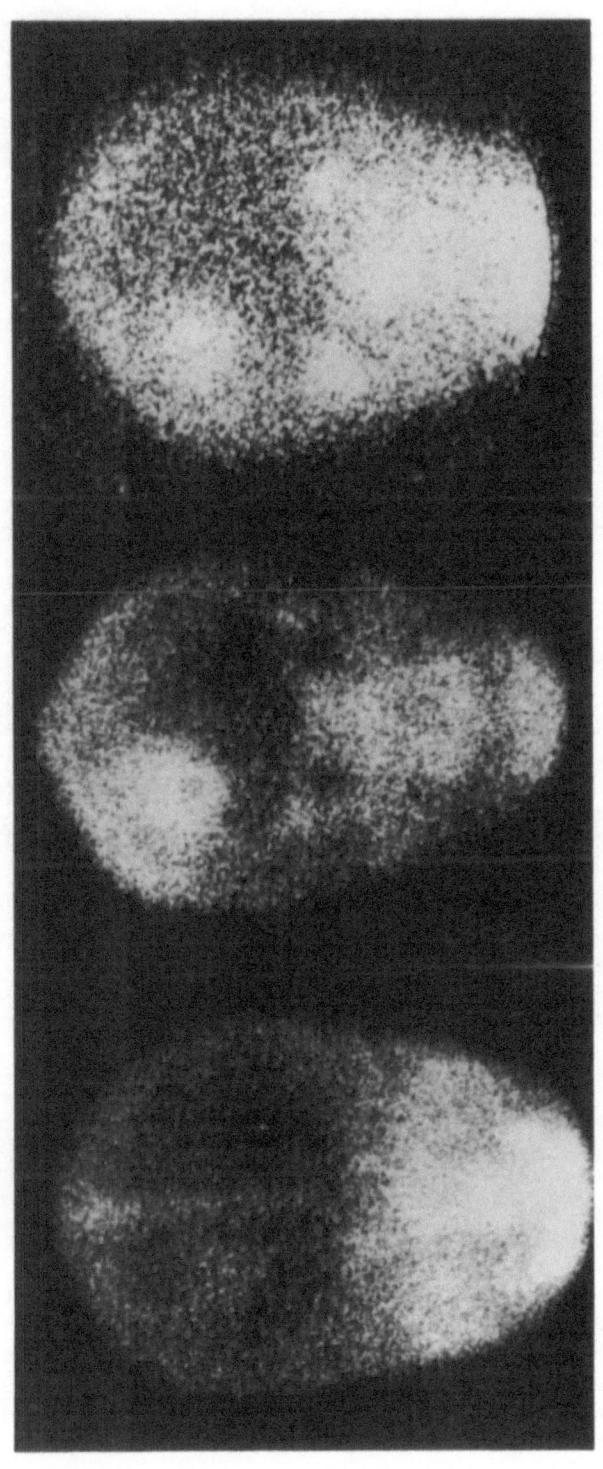

Fig. 6-9. Scintigrams utilizing 99m-Tc pertechnetate, 99m-Tc polyphosphate, and 67-Ga (left to right). Hodgkin's disease, involving the frontal bone, is demonstrated well with 99m-Tc polyphosphate and 67-Ga. Smaller lesions that are detected with 67-Ga may escape detection with a 99m-Tc pertechnetate study alone. (See Fig. 11-9).

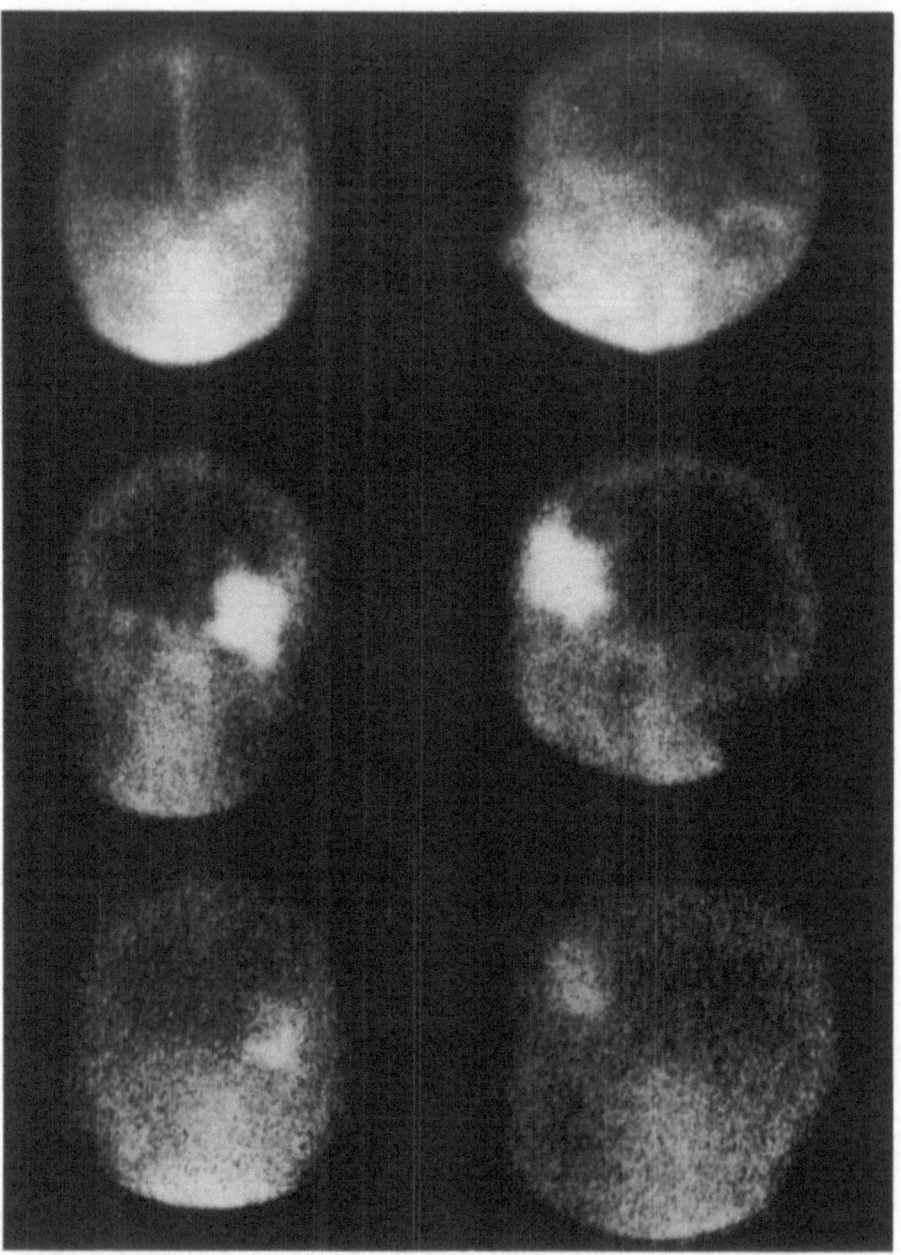

Fig. 6-10. As in Fig. 6-9 the 99m-Tc pertechnetate study (top),
while abnormal, is not nearly as clear as 99m-Tc polyphosphate
(middle), and 67-Ga (below) in demonstrating this adenocystic
carcinoma of the left lacrimal gland. Again the positive 99m-Tc
polyphosphate shows extensive involvement of the frontal bone and
defines the bony involvement more clearly than does 67-Ga.

CHAPTER 7

Tumors of the Reticuloendothelial and Hematopoietic Systems

Michael S. Milder, M. D.

Department of Nuclear Medicine, Clinical Center

National Institutes of Health, Bethesda, Maryland

Malignant Lymphomas

The localization of 67-Ga in nonosseous tumors was first observed in a patient with Hodgkin's disease (70). Since that first case, 67-Ga has been applied to the investigation of the malignant lymphomas more intensively than to any other disease. The interest in 67-Ga scintigraphy was based on the established importance of accurate staging in the management of these tumors.

It has been recognized for some time that the extent of disease at initial presentation is an important prognostic factor in Hodgkin's disease (39). In 1965 a standardized staging classification was proposed at the Rye Conference to facilitate scientific communication and provide prognostic information (40). This classification was modified at the Ann Arbor Conference in 1971 to include both clinical and pathological staging (41). Survival of patients with Hodgkin's disease correlates well with this staging system, although figures vary depending on the histological composition of the series and the manner of treatment. With application of modern radiotherapy and combination chemotherapy, the 5-year survival of patients with stage I and II disease has been improved from about 40% in earlier studies (42,43) to near 90% (44), and in stage III and IV survival has jumped from 10% (42,43) to 60-70% (44,45).

The natural history of the non-Hodgkin's lymphomas is somewhat different. They more frequently arise in extranodal tissues and quite often have disseminated to extranodal sites at the time of presentation. The usefulness of the Hodgkin's staging system has not been as thoroughly studied in the other lymphomas. However, recent reports indicate that staging of these lymphomas is also important (46).

A wide variety of clinical signs, laboratory tests and radiologic and radionuclide procedures have been employed to arrive at the clinical stage (47). All have proved to be inaccurate in an appreciable number of instances (48) although multiple abnormal tests may improve their reliability (49). As a result, laparotomy and splenectomy have been widely used to arrive at more accurate pathologic staging (48).

At the 1971 Ann Arbor Conference on Hodgkin's disease, 67-Ga scintigraphy was recognized as a promising experimental procedure (47). The experience of several groups is now available to help define the role of this approach in the staging work-up. In a series of 20 carefully staged patients, Turner and co-workers found that the 67-Ga study detected 79% of the sites of involvement (50). Kay and McCready also found a 79% true positive rate in 50 patients with Hodgkin's disease (51). The Oak Ridge Cooperative Group studied 151 untreated patients, with positive scans in 65% of the proven sites and at least one abnormality in over 90% of the patients (52). In all three studies the false positive rate was very low. No difference in accuracy was found among the four histologic types.

Thus, 20-30% of lesions may be missed by 67-Ga scintigraphy, about the same accuracy as most other diagnostic studies. However, 67-Ga scintigraphy may contribute valuable information not obtainable by other studies or even by laparotomy. All studies agree that mediastinal tumor can be detected in 85-100% of instances. This region is difficult to evaluate by other routine studies. In the abdomen, the lymphangiogram and 67-Ga scan appear complementary. Each may reveal tumor when the other may be negative or uninterpretable. However, inguinal and femoral nodes are not well evaluated by 67-Ga scintigraphy, less than 50% of the lesions being detected.

The 67-Ga scan may be the only means of detecting extranodal disease. Bone, lung, brain and other metastases may appear on the 67-Ga scan before conventional studies can detect them. This information is of great importance in planning proper therapy for the patient.

Experience with non-Hodgkin's lymphomas is limited to the Cooperative Group Report on 167 cases (53). The scan was positive in 51% of the proven sites of involvement. Accuracy was highly correlated with histology and varied with the concentration of histiocytes. Thus, histiocytic lymphoma was detected in over 70% of the sites, mixed histiocytic-lymphocytic type in over 50%, and lymphocytic lymphoma in about 35% of sites as in Hodgkin's disease, where mediastinal adenopathy was most reliably detected.

Because of the high incidence of stage IV disease, 67-Ga scintigraphy may prove more valuable in evaluation of the non-Hodgkin's lymphomas than in Hodgkin's disease. Particularly in histiocytic lymphoma, where accuracy equals that in Hodgkin's disease, the ability of the 67-Ga scan to find disseminated disease should prove helpful.

Aside from staging, 67-Ga may have other roles in the evaluation of lymphomas. 67-Ga uptake may be an independent indicator of tumor response to therapy. Many reports cite the disappearance of 67-Ga uptake with treatment, but proper long-term studies in lymphomas have not been done. Similarly, 67-Ga scintigraphy may offer a method for following up to detect relapse. Because of the low incidence of false positives, a focus of 67-Ga activity usually indicates tumor.

Leukemia

Staging the anatomical extent of disease is not a major concern in the leukemias. All types are considered to be systemic malignancies from the time of presentation. The neoplasm can be identified and followed easily by bone marrow examination. There is usually no need to locate occult sites of disease.

For these reasons, 67-Ga scintigraphy has not been used in the evaluation of leukemia at most centers. However, the 67-Ga scan does provide a distinctive pattern and may be clinically useful in evaluating some of the complications of the leukemias (38).

The typical 67-Ga scan pattern in untreated acute leukemia is an increase in activity in the marrow of the entire skeleton. This is most apparent around the large joints and in the shafts of the femurs. The pattern can be seen in both acute myelocytic (AML) and acute lymphocytic leukemia (ALL). In leukemic children bone uptake may exceed the usual prominent activity seen in growing bones.

Bone marrow uptake is related to the percentage of blast cells in the bone marrow. When 80% or more of the marrow cells are blasts, over 75% of patients show abnormal 67-Ga concentration in the bone marrow. At lower degrees of infiltration, this pattern is uncommon.

Bone uptake may be prominent in chronic myelogenous leukemia (CML), especially when these patients develop blast crisis. In contrast, chronic lymphocytic leukemia (CLL) usually presents an entirely normal scan.

Increased bone uptake is not specific for leukemia. It may be seen in any other tumor invading the bone marrow. In addition, in the lymphomas abnormal bone uptake may be observed in the presence of a normal marrow biopsy. It is not known whether this represents a pre-malignant state or a non-specific inflammatory change such as occurs in the liver in Hodgkin's disease.

In addition to osseous activity, an enlarged liver and spleen may be seen on the 67-Ga scan. Splenomegaly is greatest and splenic uptake most avid in CML, where spleen activity may obscure most of the abdomen. Splenic infarction may be detected by irregularities or changes in the splenic image.

Focal leukemic disease is often seen in AML or CML in the form of myeloblastomas or chloromas. These masses of myeloblasts also accumulate 67-Ga and may be visualized and followed until their resolution by scanning. Focal leukemic infiltrates may be observed in the testes, breasts, nasopharynx and other regions.

Patients with leukemia are particularly susceptible to infectious complications, and 67-Ga scintigraphy may play a role in the investigation of fevers and the evaluation of abscesses (see Chapter 12).

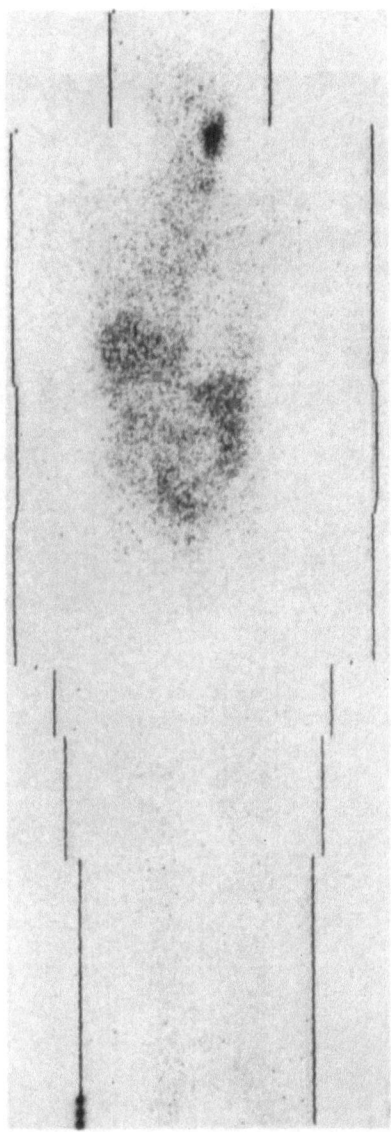

Fig. 7-1. Hodgkin's disease - Stage I: A 75-year-old man had a
6-month history of left cervical adenopathy. Two months prior to
this scan, a mass was discovered invading the left maxillary sinus
which was excised. On admission, he had a 4 cm left posterior cervical node and several smaller nodes on the left neck. Biopsy of
these revealed Hodgkin's disease with mixed cellularity (Lennert's
type). The 67-Ga scan shows prominent uptake in the left cervical
area corresponding to the clinically suspected nodes. There is some
bowel localization of 67-Ga. All other studies were normal. The
patient was stage 1E because of extension into the maxillary sinus.

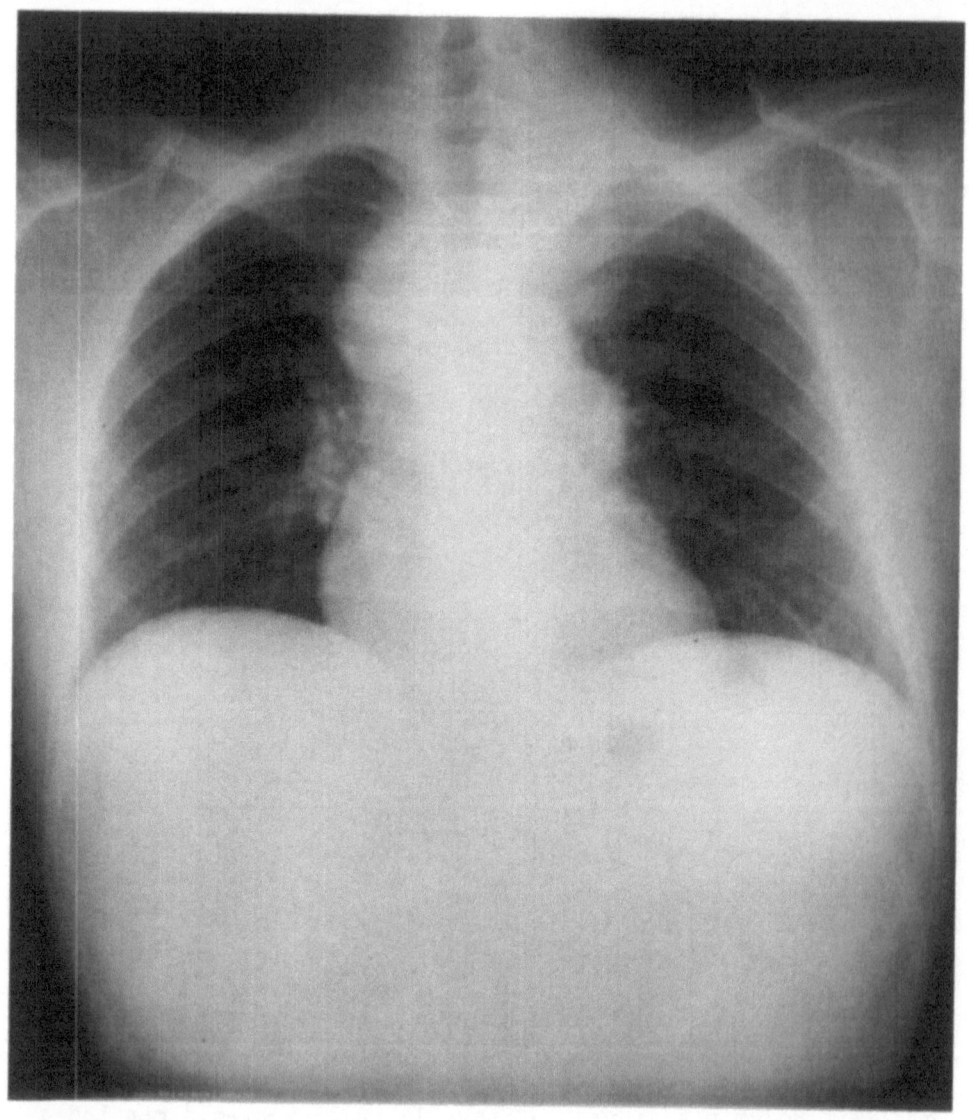

Fig. 7-2A. Hodgkin's disease - Stage II: A 31-year-old man had a
one-year history of a left cervical mass followed by pruritus,
fever and a 20-lb. weight loss. On admission he had palpable
adenopathy in the left cervical and supraclavicular areas and both
axillae. The chest radiograph reveals marked mediastinal and
hilar adenopathy.

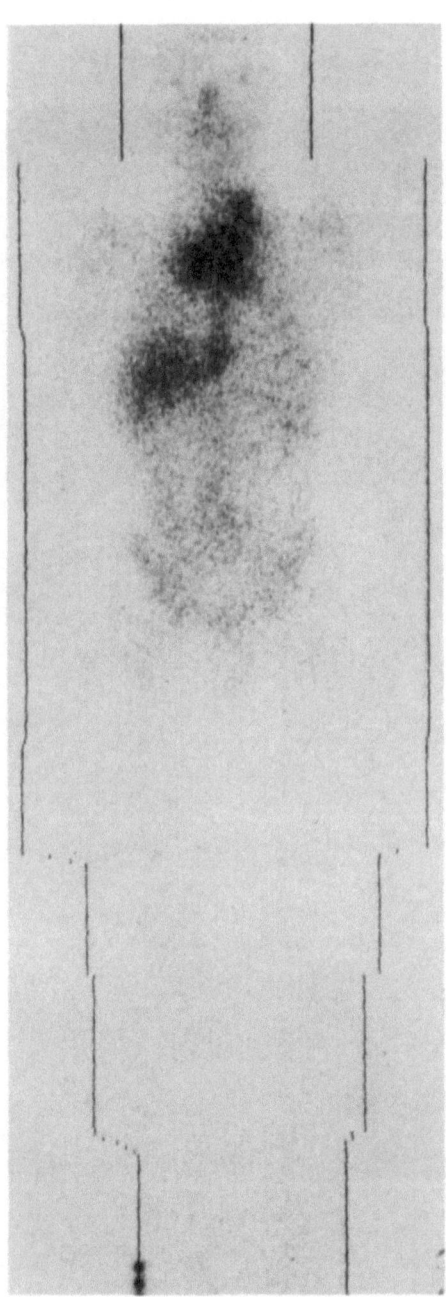

Fig. 7-2B. Hodgkin's disease - Stage II (continued): This 67-Ga
scan confirms the presence of tumor in the left supraclavicular
area and mediastinum. The lymphangiogram was equivocal and peritoneoscopy yielded normal liver biopsies. Biopsy of a neck node
revealed Hodgkin's disease, nodular sclerosis type.

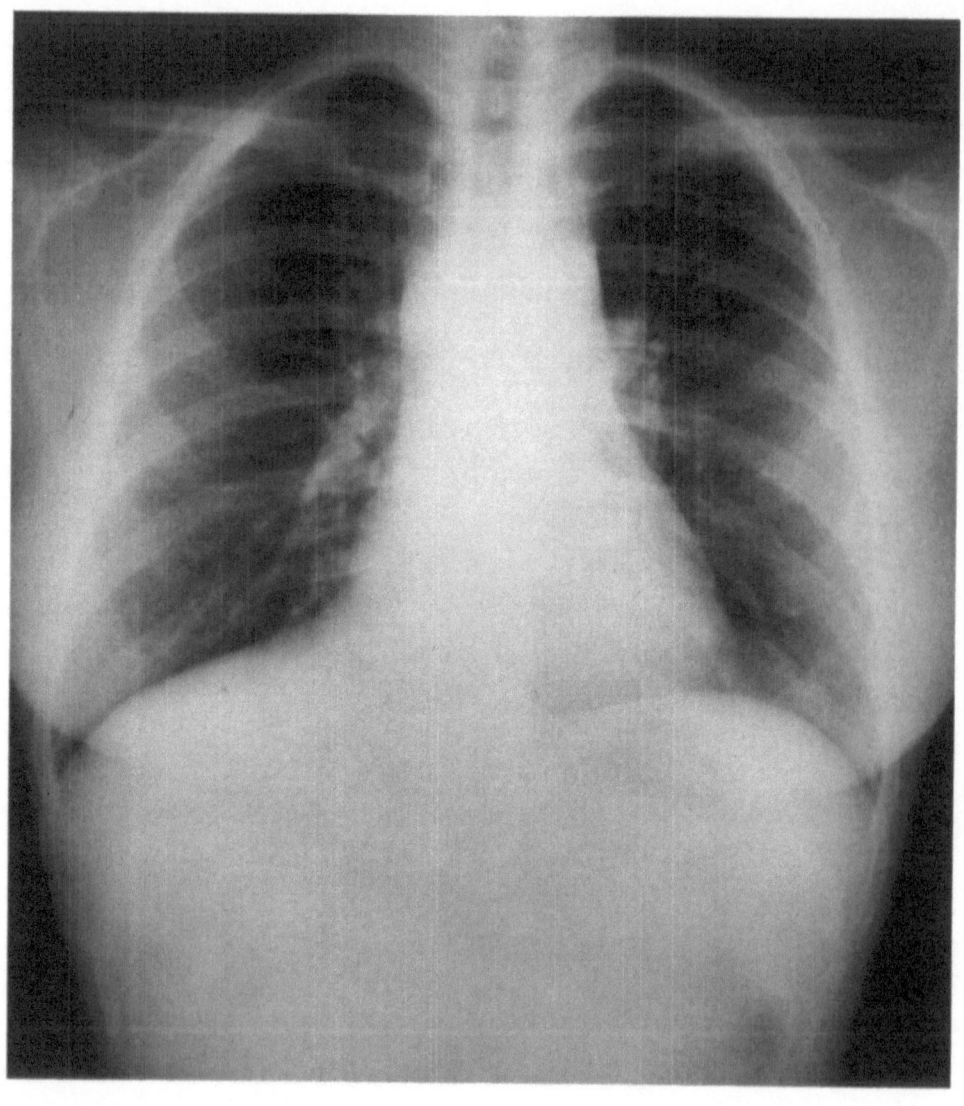

Fig. 7-3A. Hodgkin's disease - Stage II: A 22-year-old woman
noticed a left axillary lump three months prior to study by scan.
She later developed cough, dyspnea, orthopnea, fevers, sweats, and
anorexia. Physical examination showed bilateral cervical, axillary
and left supraclavicular adenopathy. The chest film shows slight
mediastinal widening and prominent hila.

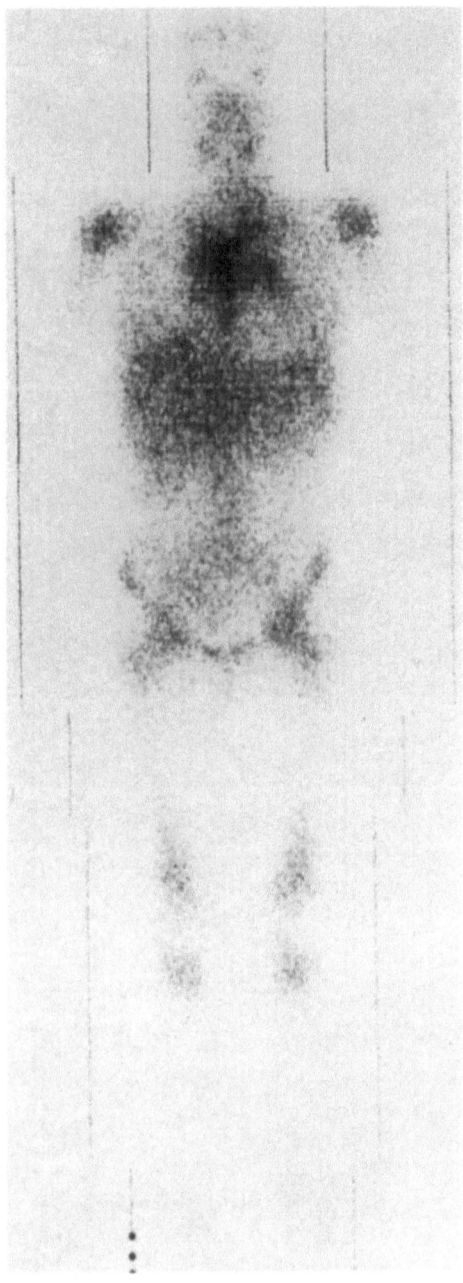

Fig. 7-3B. Hodgkin's disease – Stage II (continued): The 67-Ga study unequivocally reveals mediastinal, hilar, cervical and left supraclavicular uptake. Lymphangiogram, bone marrow and liver biopsies were normal. Biopsy of a left axillary node revealed Hodgkin's disease, nodular sclerosis type.

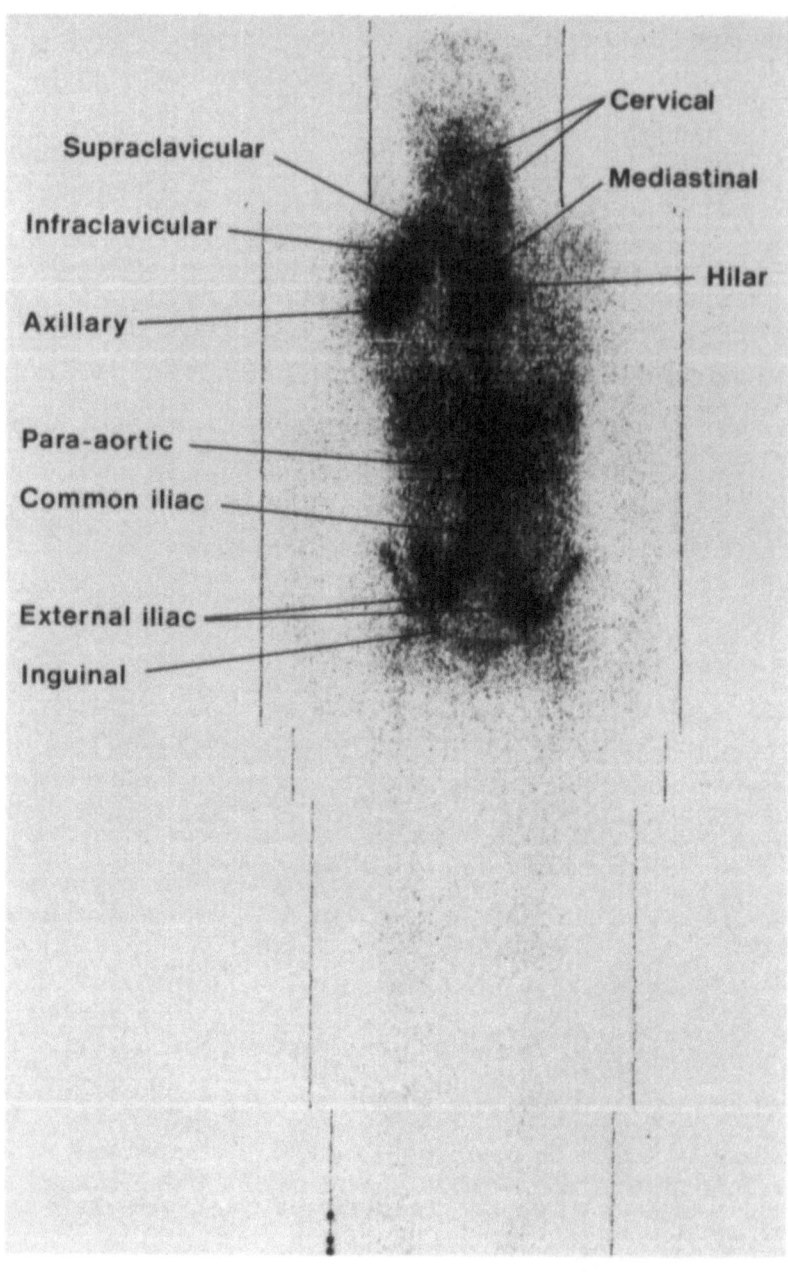

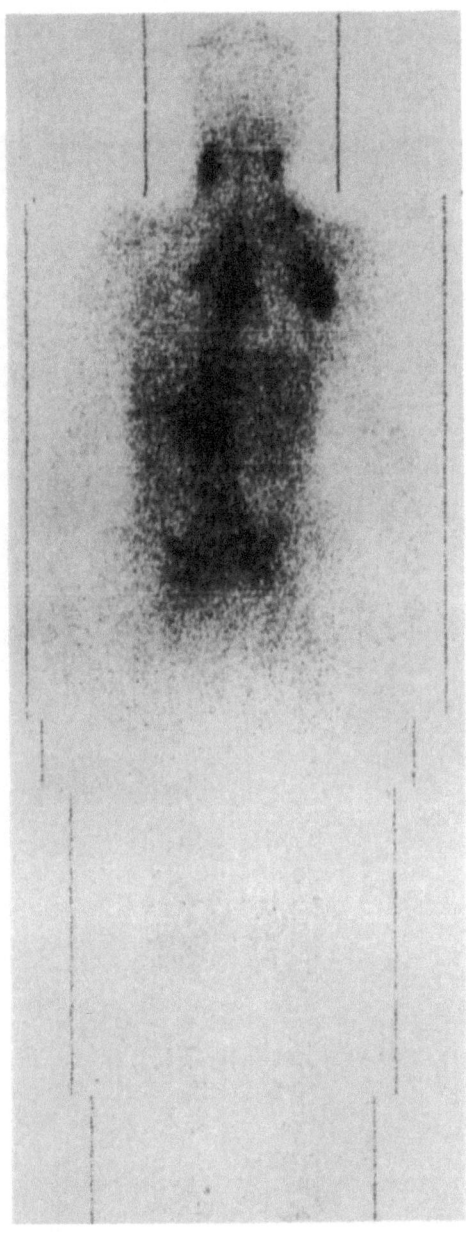

Fig. 7-4. Hodgkin's disease - Stage III: A 25-year-old woman presented with generalized adenopathy, fever, and weight loss. Biopsy of a cervical node showed Hodgkin's disease, nodular sclerosing type. Chest film and lymphangiogram showed abnormal lymph nodes. Anterior and posterior 67-Ga scans reveal abnormal uptake in all major lymph node groups bilaterally. Biopsies of liver and bone marrow were normal.

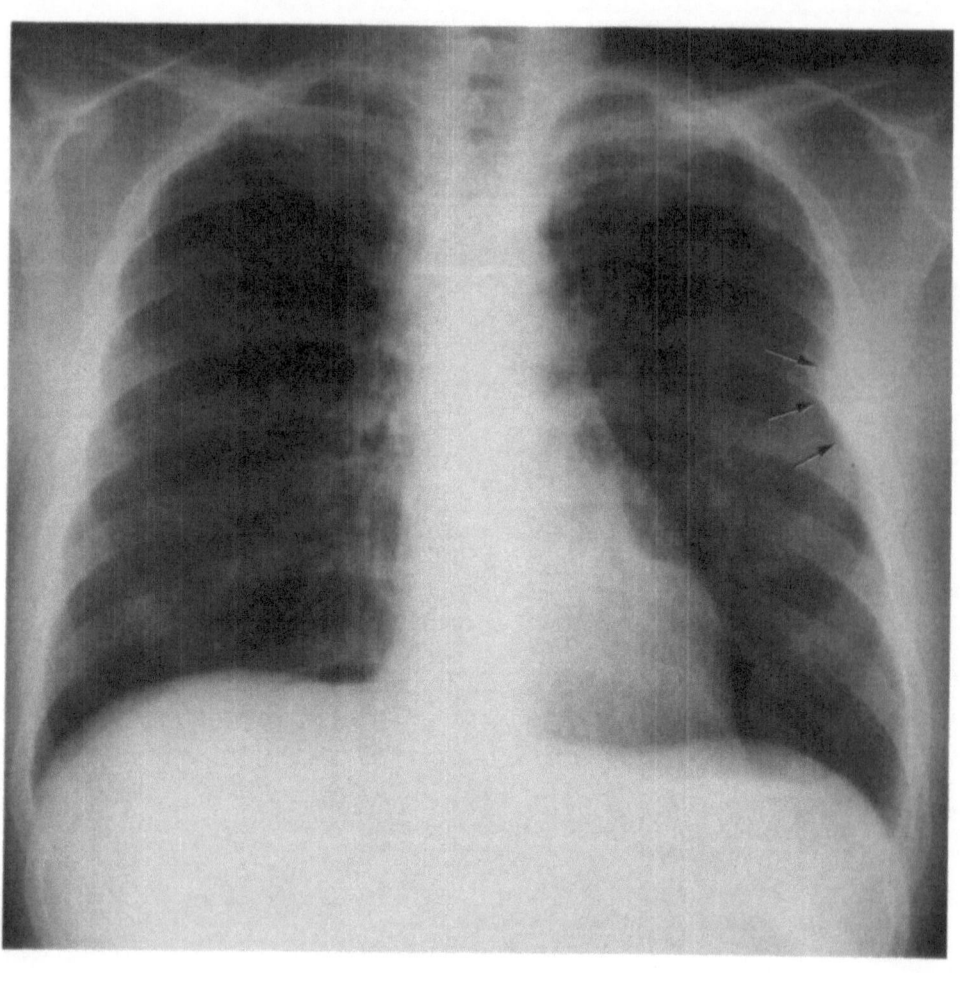

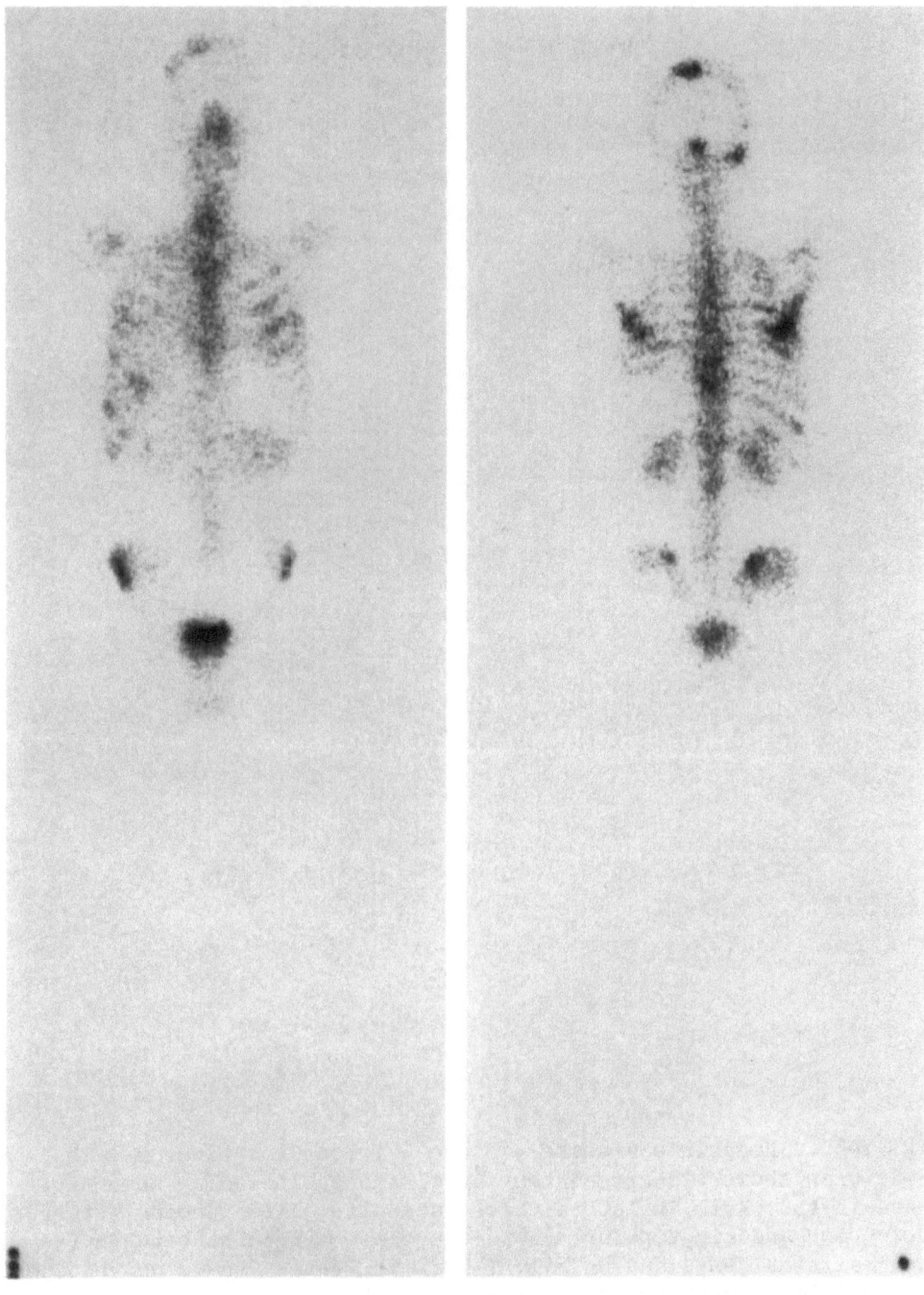

Fig. 7-5B. Hodgkin's disease - Stage IV, Bone (continued):
99m-Tc-polyphosphate bone scan indicates widespread bony involvement.

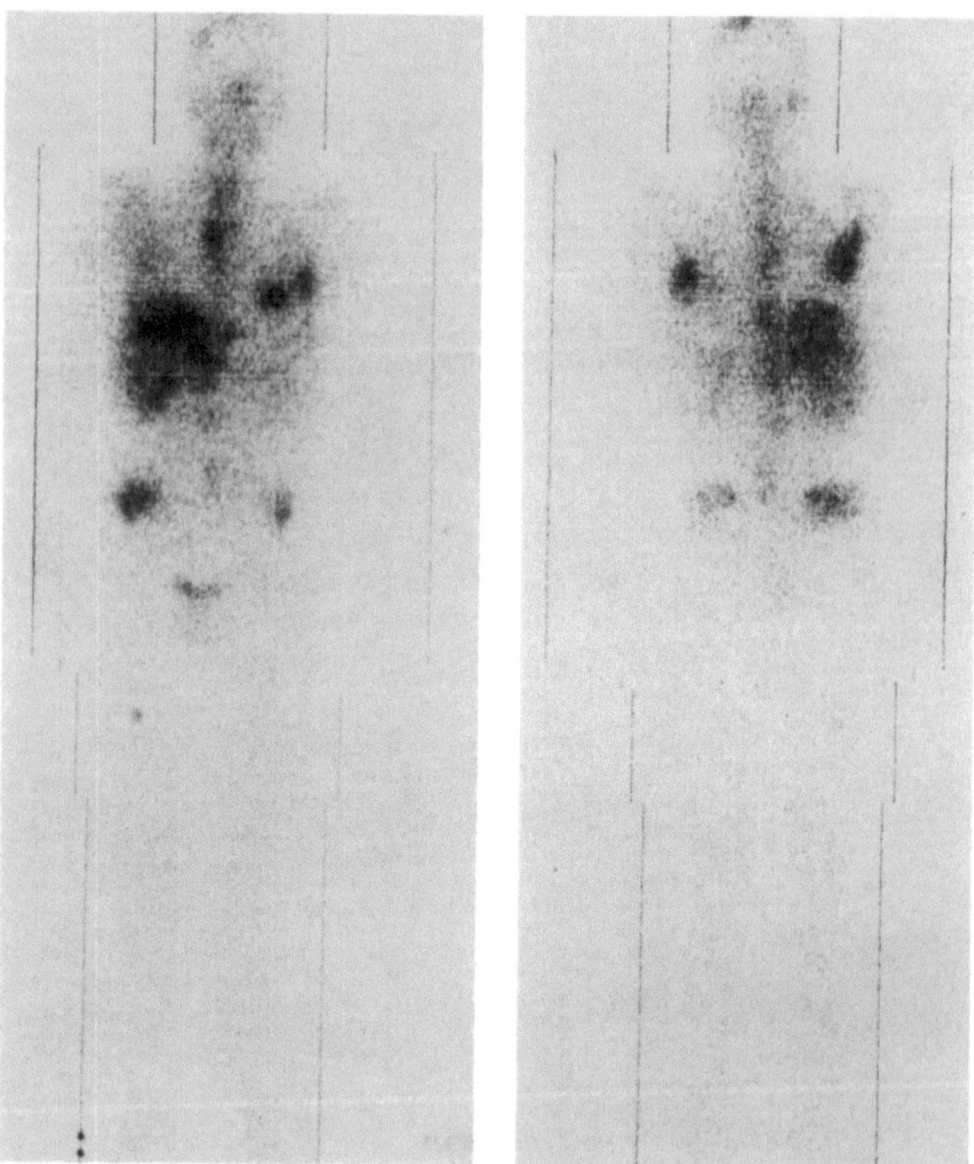

Fig. 7-5C. Hodgkin's disease - Stage IV, Bone (continued): The
67-Ga scan shows widespread bony involvement, including several
areas in the skull, bilateral ribs, scapulae, iliac crests, sternum,
pubic bone and right femur. Note the close agreement between the
abnormalities above and in Fig. 7-5B. While the 99m-Tc polyphosphate
scan provides superior resolution, many of the lesions show greater
activity on the 67-Ga scan. Because of these studies tomography
was performed (Fig. 7-5D), revealing a destructive lesion in the
left 5th rib. A needle biopsy yielded Reed-Sternberg cells.

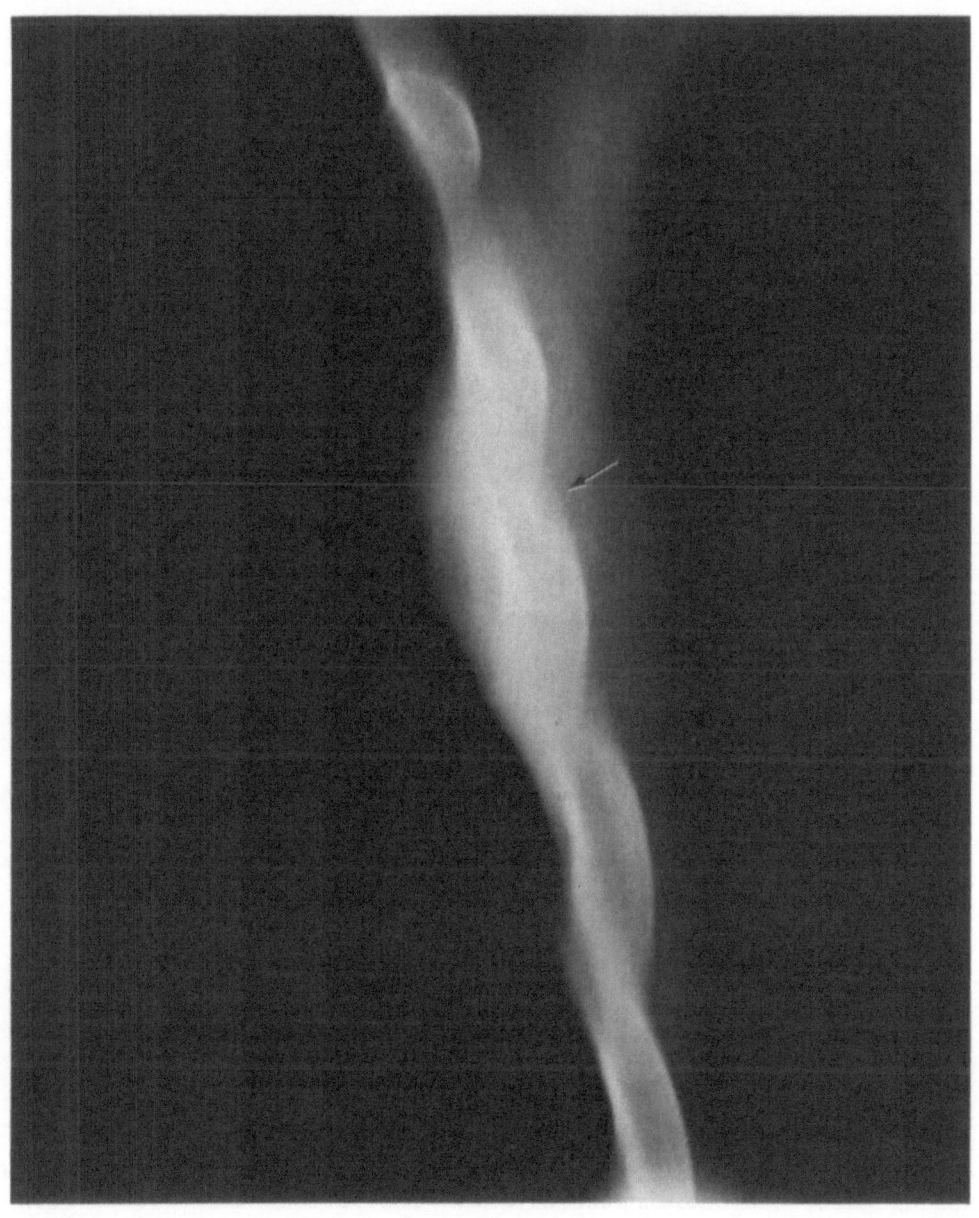

Fig. 7-5D (continued)

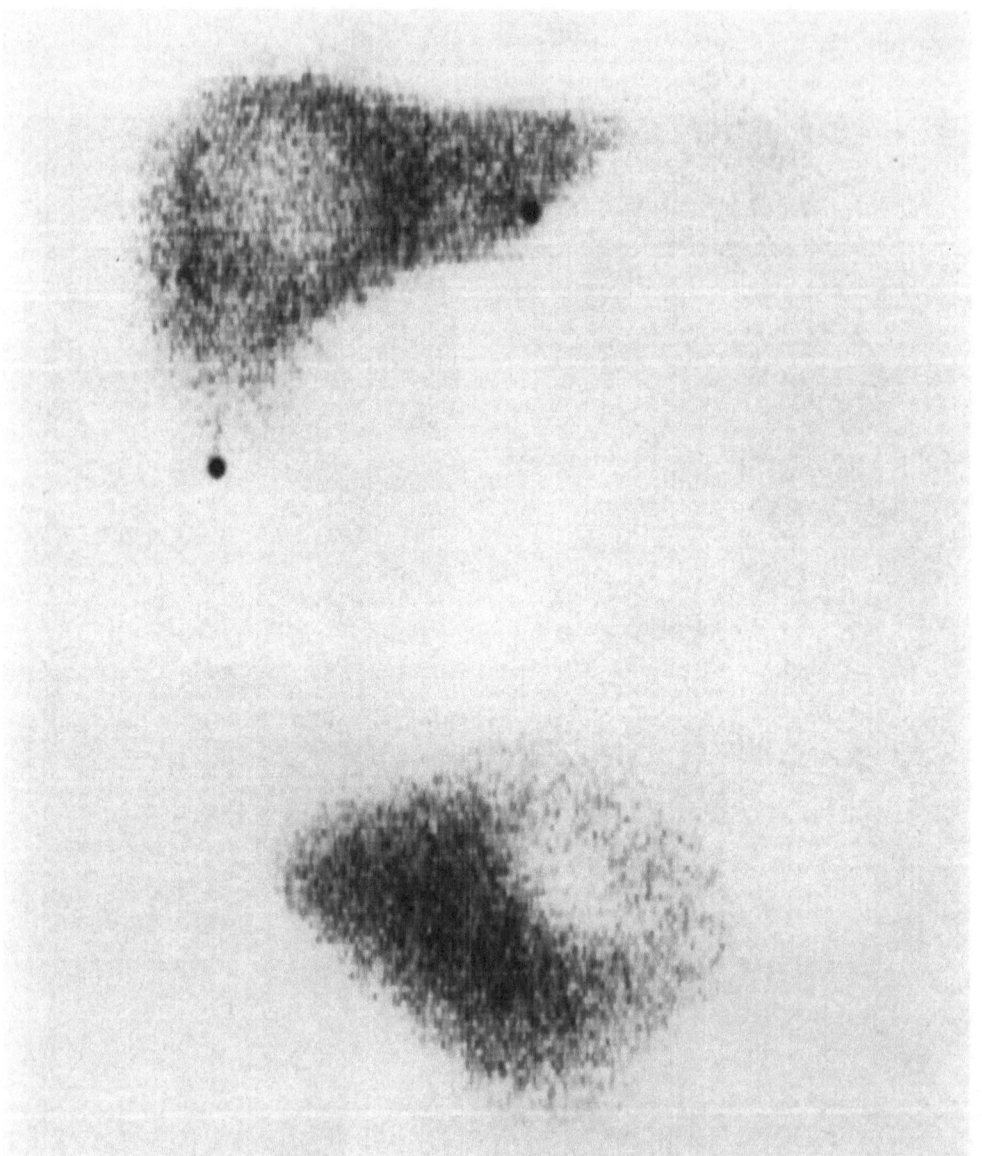

Fig. 7-6A. Malignant Lymphoma, lymphocytic, well differentiated, diffuse - Stage IV, Liver: Six months prior to admission this 64-year-old man became jaundiced and a hepatic mass was found which was diagnosed as cholangiocarcinoma. The patient was treated with 5-fluorouracil and irradiation. Four months later left axillary adenopathy appeared and lymphoma was found on biopsy. An upper gastrointestinal series revealed an ulceration in the stomach. A large filling defect is seen on this 99m-Tc sulfur colloid liver scan with a smaller defect at the lower edge of the right lobe.

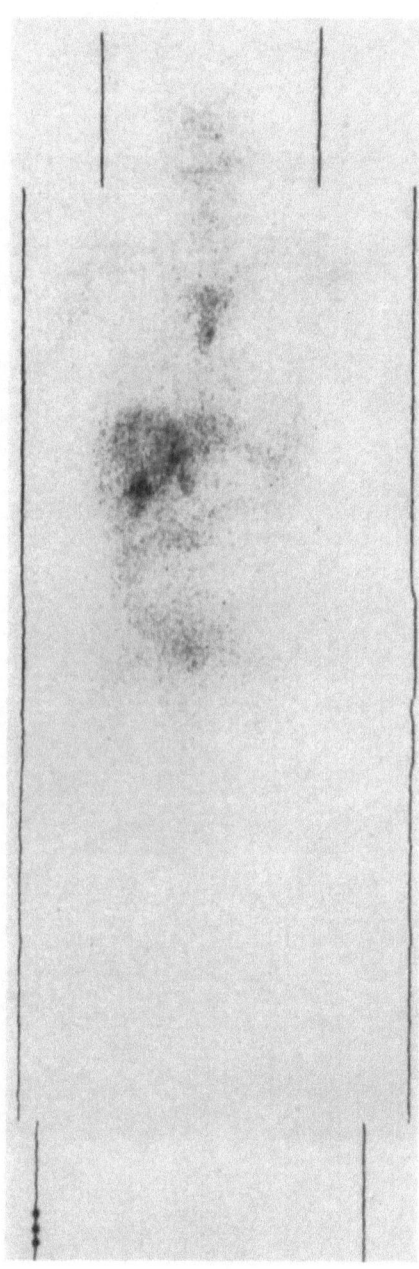

Fig. 7-6B. Malignant Lymphoma, lymphocytic, well differentiated, diffuse - Stage IV, Liver (continued): The 67-Ga scan shows uptake in this smaller area of abnormality and in the epigastrium and sternum. A bone marrow biopsy showed replacement by lymphoma. The patient deteriorated rapidly and died two months later. At autopsy, lymphoma was found in the liver, stomach and bone marrow.

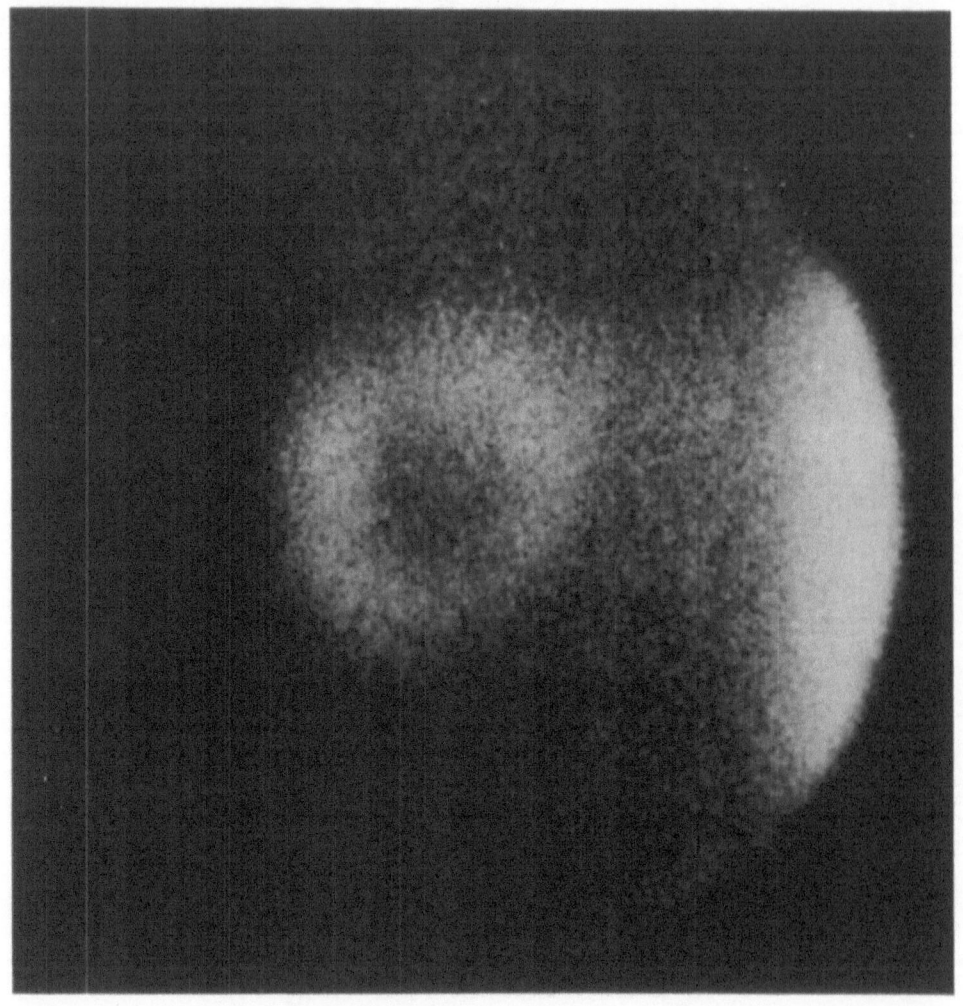

Fig. 7-7A. Malignant Lymphoma, mixed histiocytic-lymphocytic -
Stage III, Spleen: A 56-year-old woman had a one-year history of
right cervical adenopathy. Biopsy of this area showed lymphoma.
A lymphangiogram was positive. This 99m-Tc sulfur colloid liver-
spleen scan shows a large central filling defect in the spleen.

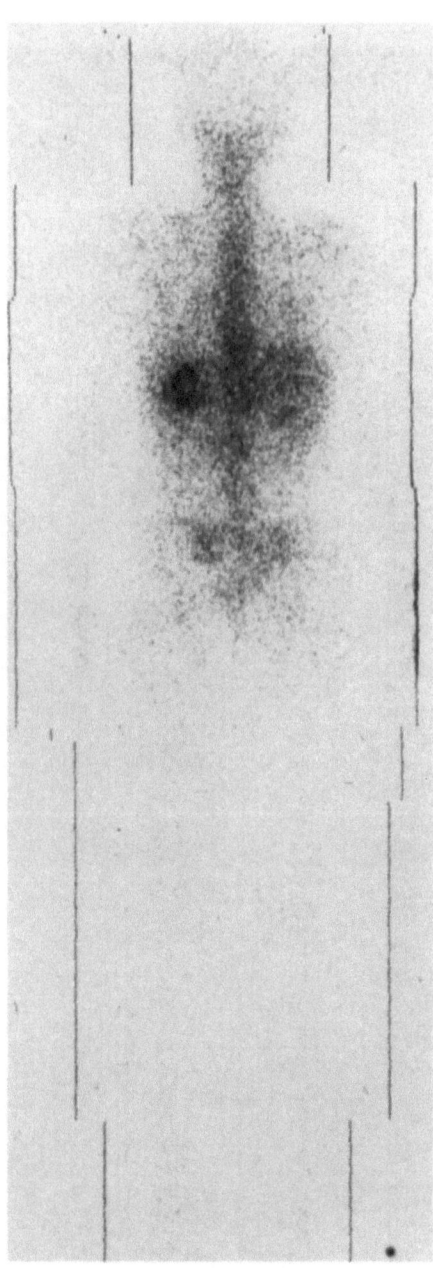

Fig. 7-7B. Malignant Lymphoma, mixed histiocytic-lymphocytic –
Stage III, Spleen (continued): The 67-Ga scan reveals increased
uptake in the center of the spleen on the posterior view. After
splenectomy the spleen was found to have a large central tumor
mass. The 67-Ga study complemented the spleen scan by limiting
the differential diagnosis of a filling defect to tumor or abscess.

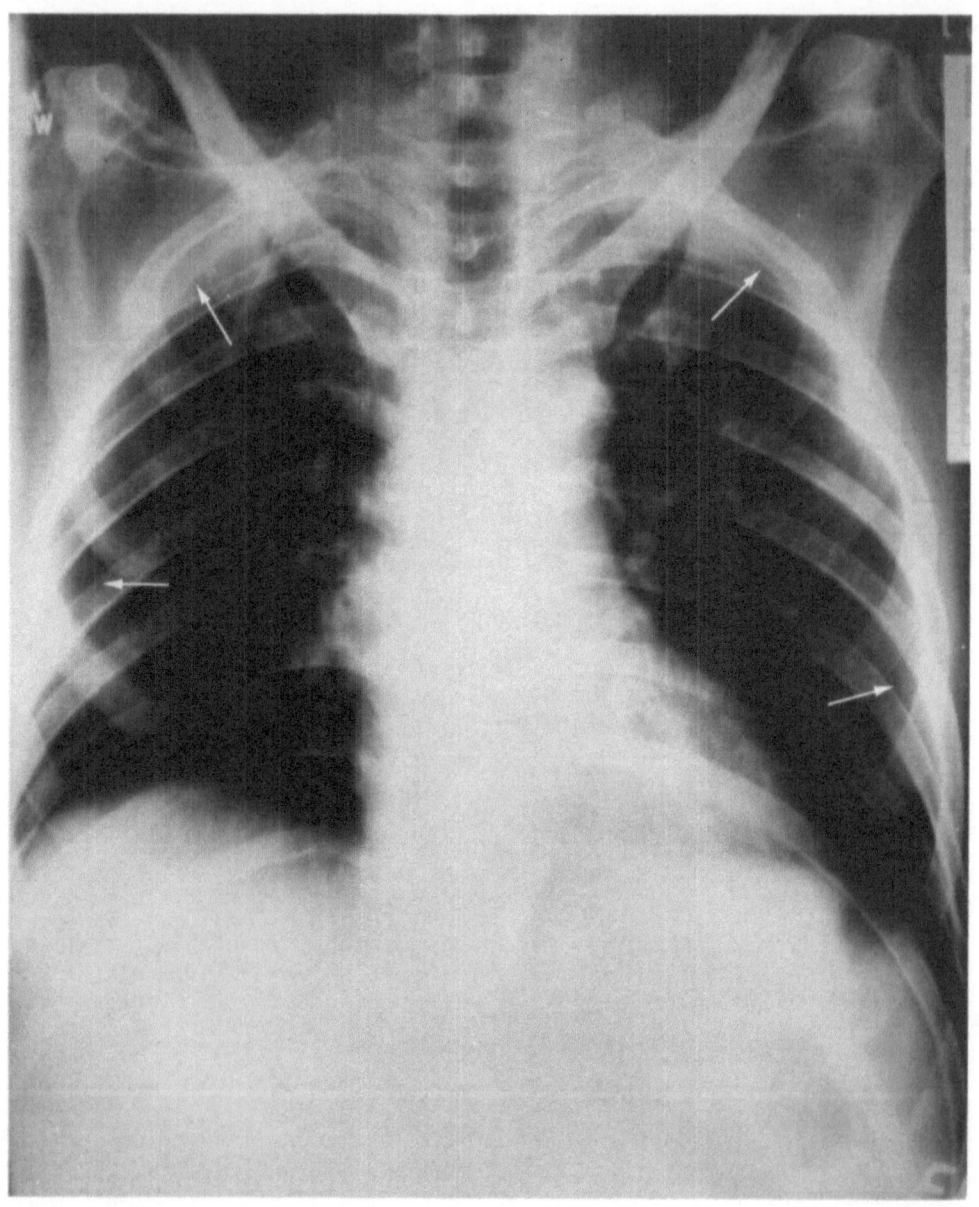

Fig. 7-8A. Malignant Lymphoma, histiocytic, diffuse - Stage IV,
Bone and Pleura: A 54-year-old man presented with inguinal
adenopathy. Biopsy of a left inguinal node showed lymphoma. The
chest x-ray indicates some apical and lateral pleural thickening
(arrows) thought to be related to inactive tuberculosis. Mediastinal and hilar adenopathy was also noted.

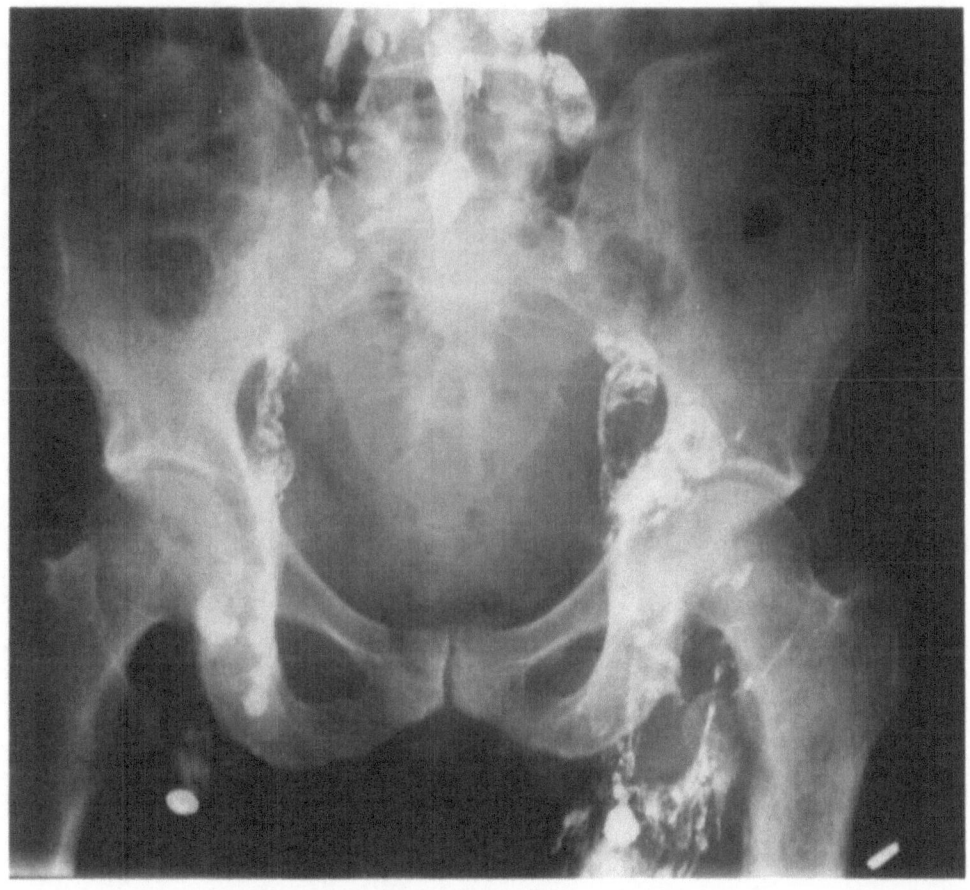

Fig. 7-8B. Malignant Lymphoma, histiocytic, diffuse - Stage IV,
Bone and Pleura (continued): The lymphangiogram shows abnormalities
of the paraaortic, iliac, and inguinal nodes. Note also the
destructive process in the left femur with pathologic fracture of
the lesser trochanter.

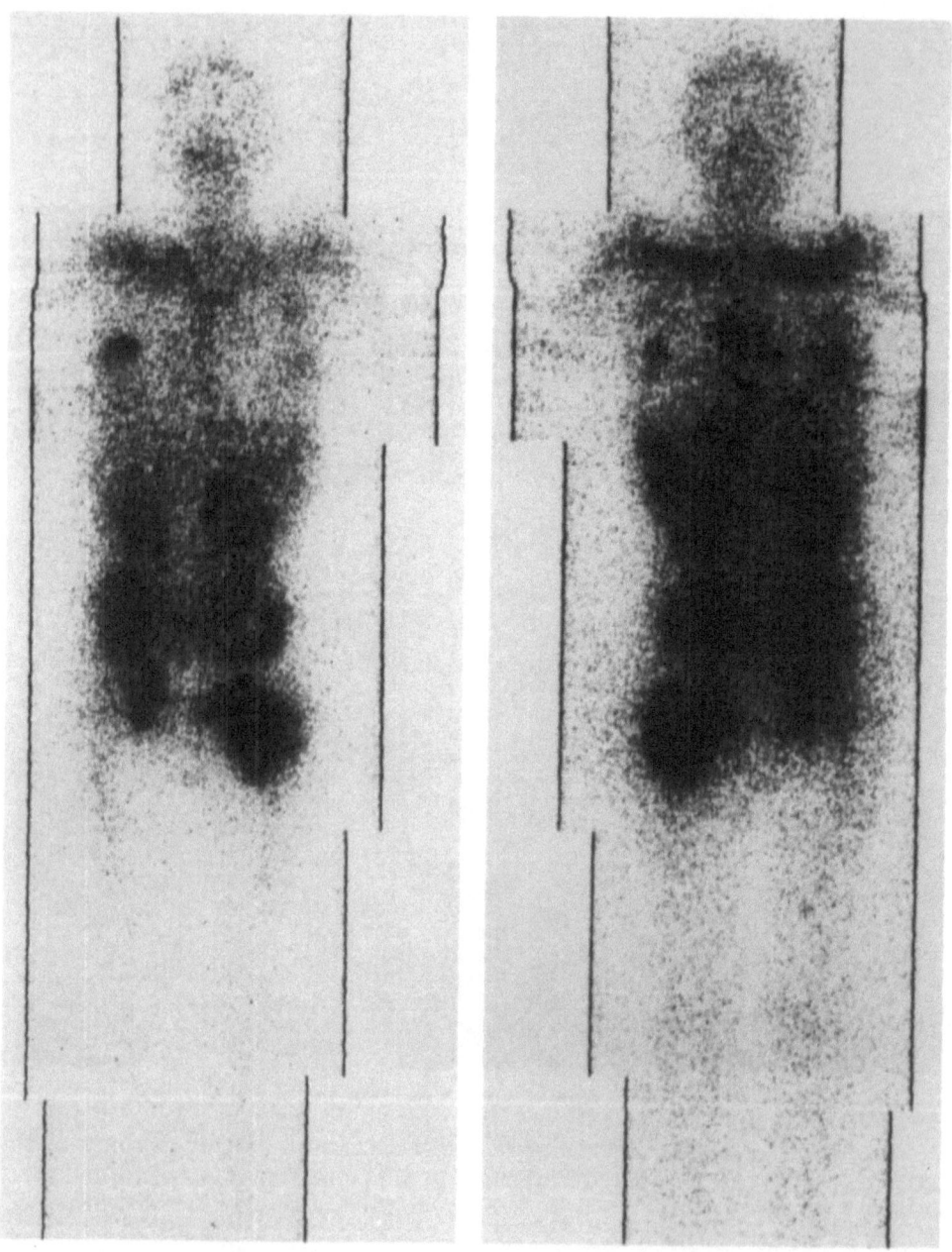

Fig. 7-8C. Malignant Lymphoma, histiocytic, diffuse - Stage IV,
Bone and Pleura (continued): The 67-Ga study shows intense uptake
in the left femur, pelvic bones, and iliac and inguinal nodes.
The kidneys also appear to be involved. In the chest there is
67-Ga activity in the areas of pleural thickening, indicating
pleural involvement by lymphoma.

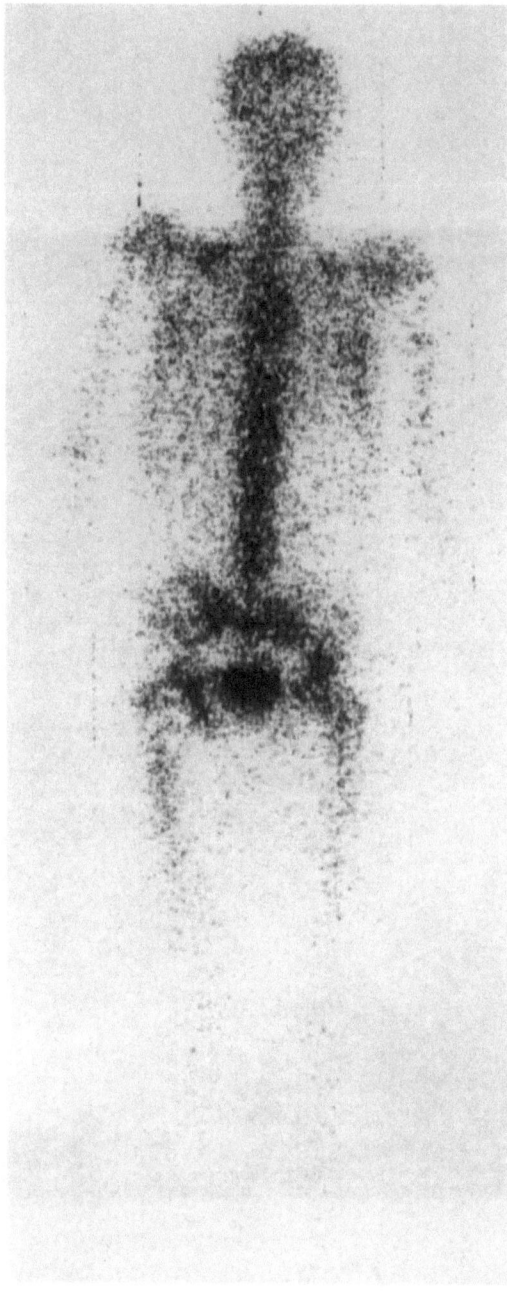

Fig. 7-8D. Malignant Lymphoma, histiocytic, diffuse – Stage IV, Bone and Pleura (continued): An 18-Fluorine bone scan showed no uptake in the femur. Biopsy of this lesion showed only necrotic tumor.

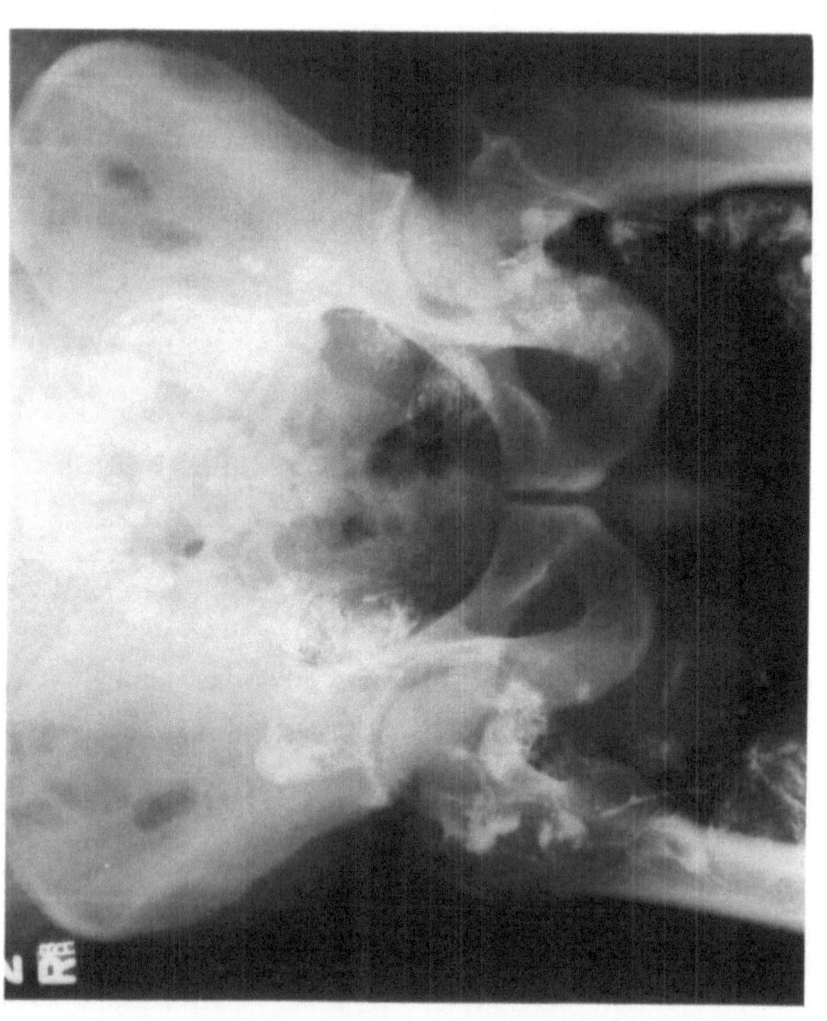

Fig. 7-9A. Malignant Lymphoma, histiocytic – correlation with lymphangiogram: A 38-year-old man presented with a one-year history of cervical adenopathy and wheezing. Biopsies of cervical and inguinal nodes showed lymphoma. A chest x-ray revealed massive hilar adenopathy which was irradiated for relief of the patient's dyspnea. A subsequent lymphangiogram shows abdominal and iliac nodes up to 10 cm in size.

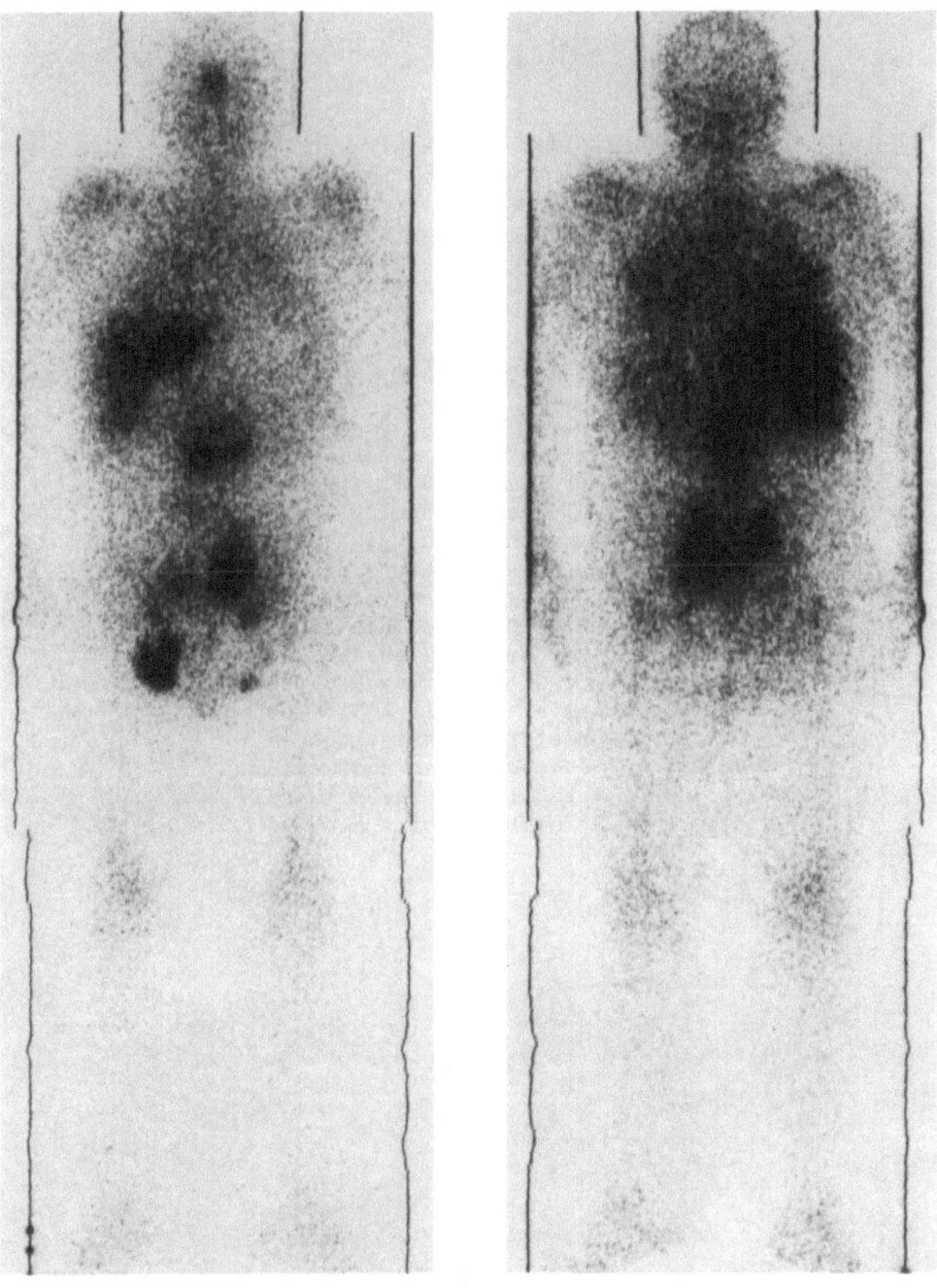

Fig. 7-9B. Malignant Lymphoma, histiocytic – correlation with lymphangiogram (continued): The 67-Ga scan indicates large accumulations of 67-Ga in the paraortic, iliac and inguinal areas. Note that the previously irradiated mediastinum appears normal.

Fig. 7-10. Malignant Lymphoma, undifferentiated - Stage IV, Soft Tissue:
Lymphoma was diagnosed three years
before admission on biopsy of a left
breast mass in this 43-year old woman.
Her bone marrow was also involved. She
achieved a remission on combination
chemotherapy which lasted three years.
Then she developed soft-tissue masses
in the left ankle and calf. A 67-Ga
scan shows three distinct lesions in
the left leg. A bone scan and marrow
biopsy were normal. All three masses
subsided with local radiotherapy.

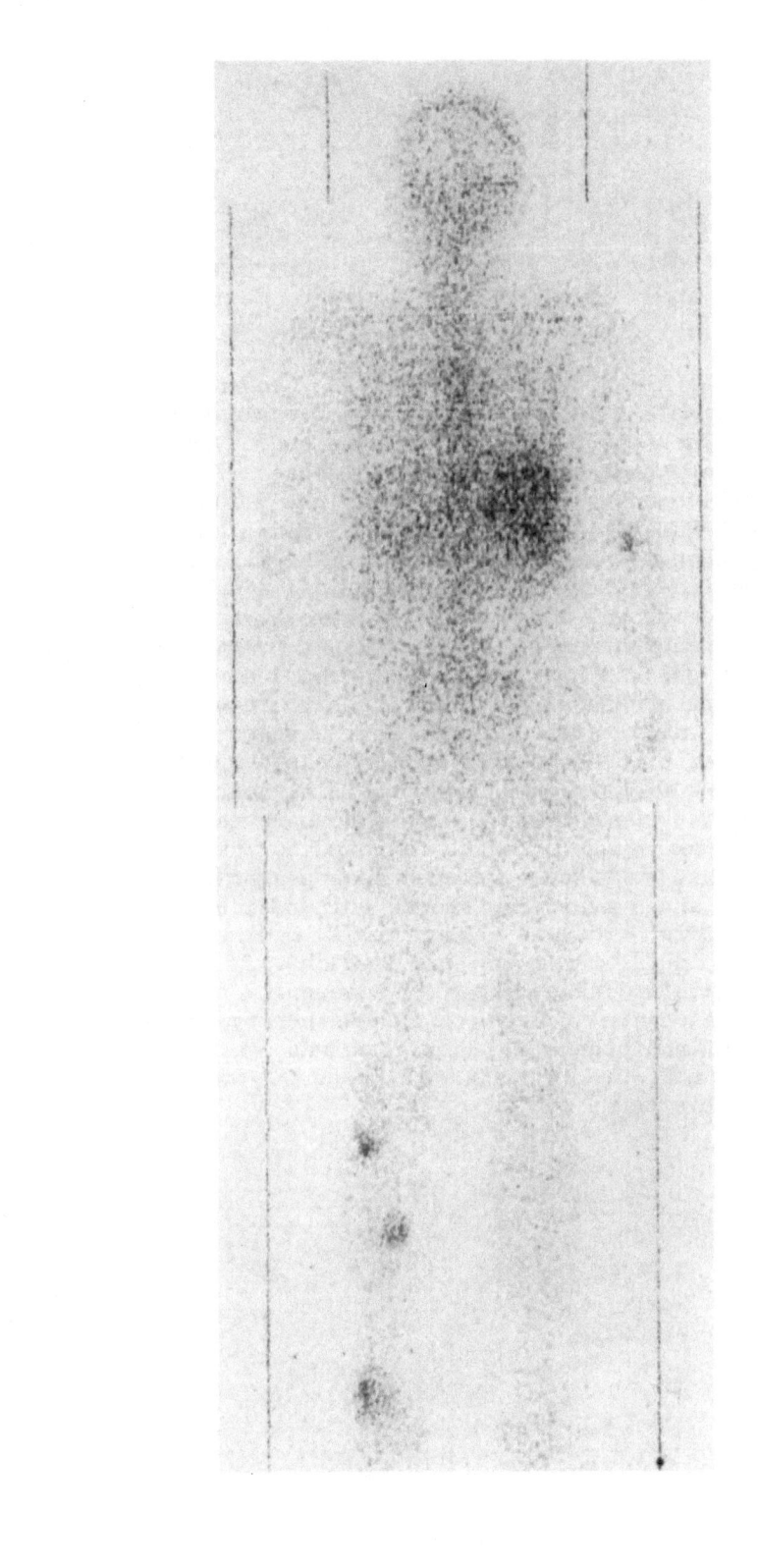

Fig. 7-11A. Hodgkin's disease - Sequential
Studies: A 17-year-old male was evaluated
for back pain. A biopsy of the second lumbar
vertebra revealed Hodgkin's disease. Further
involvement was found in the right ilium,
left humerus, and left cervical node, and a
lymphangiogram was abnormal. The patient
had fevers, sweats and weight loss. A
remission was achieved with chemotherapy
and radiotherapy. One year later he returned
with pain in his right shoulder and chest
and recurrent sweats. Although there were
no physical signs of recurrent disease, this
posterior 67-Ga scan shows increased uptake
in the right ilium and sacro-iliac joint
and the upper spine. A bone scan revealed
the same areas. He was followed for two
months, but then developed weakness of the
legs and a myelogram showed compression at
the first thoracic vertebra. At laminectomy
an epidural tumor was found which was
Hodgkin's disease, nodular sclerosing type.
He was again treated with chemotherapy and
local radiotherapy. Remission was again
achieved. (Note that this posterior view
is reversed.)

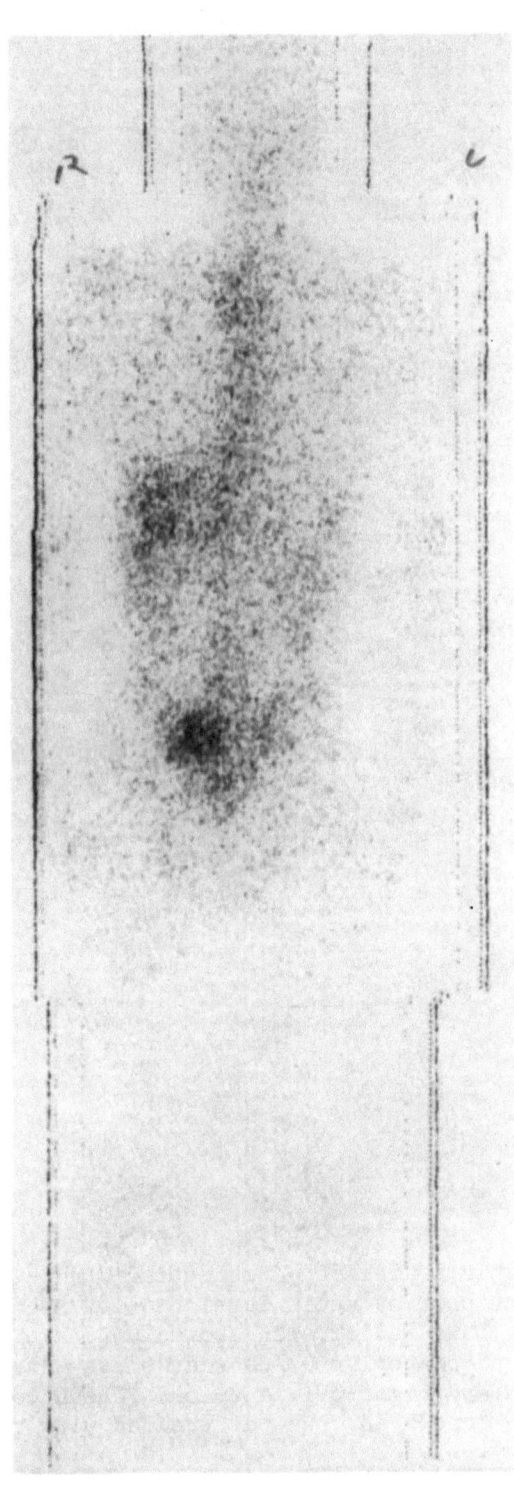

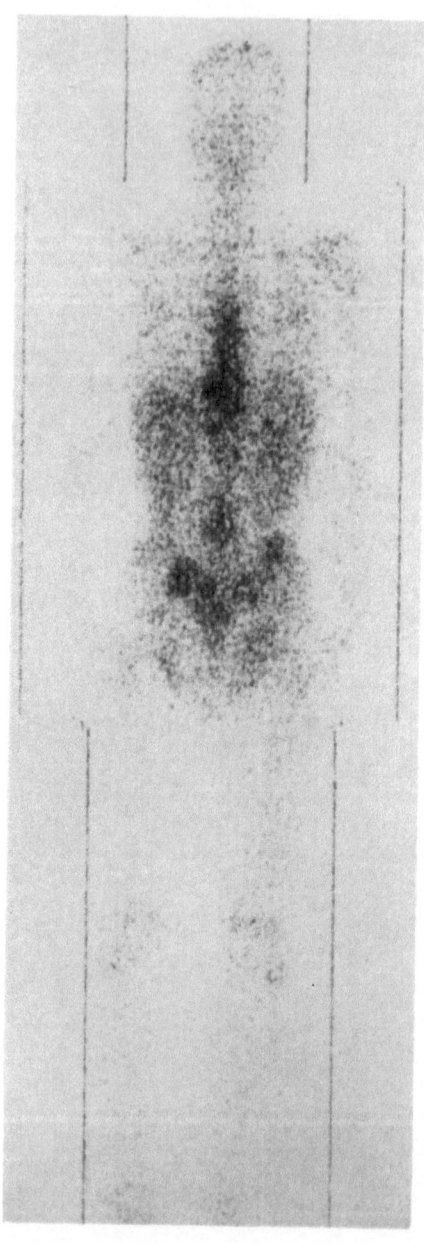

Fig. 7-11B. Hodgkin's disease - Sequential Studies (continued):
One year later the patient again developed low back pain, fever
and weight loss. Bone radiographs showed a paravertebral mass at
T9-11. This second posterior 67-Ga scan shows thoracic and lumbar
spine involvement and right pelvic tumor. These bony abnormalities
were confirmed on bone scan. He was treated with vinblastine and
local radiotherapy.

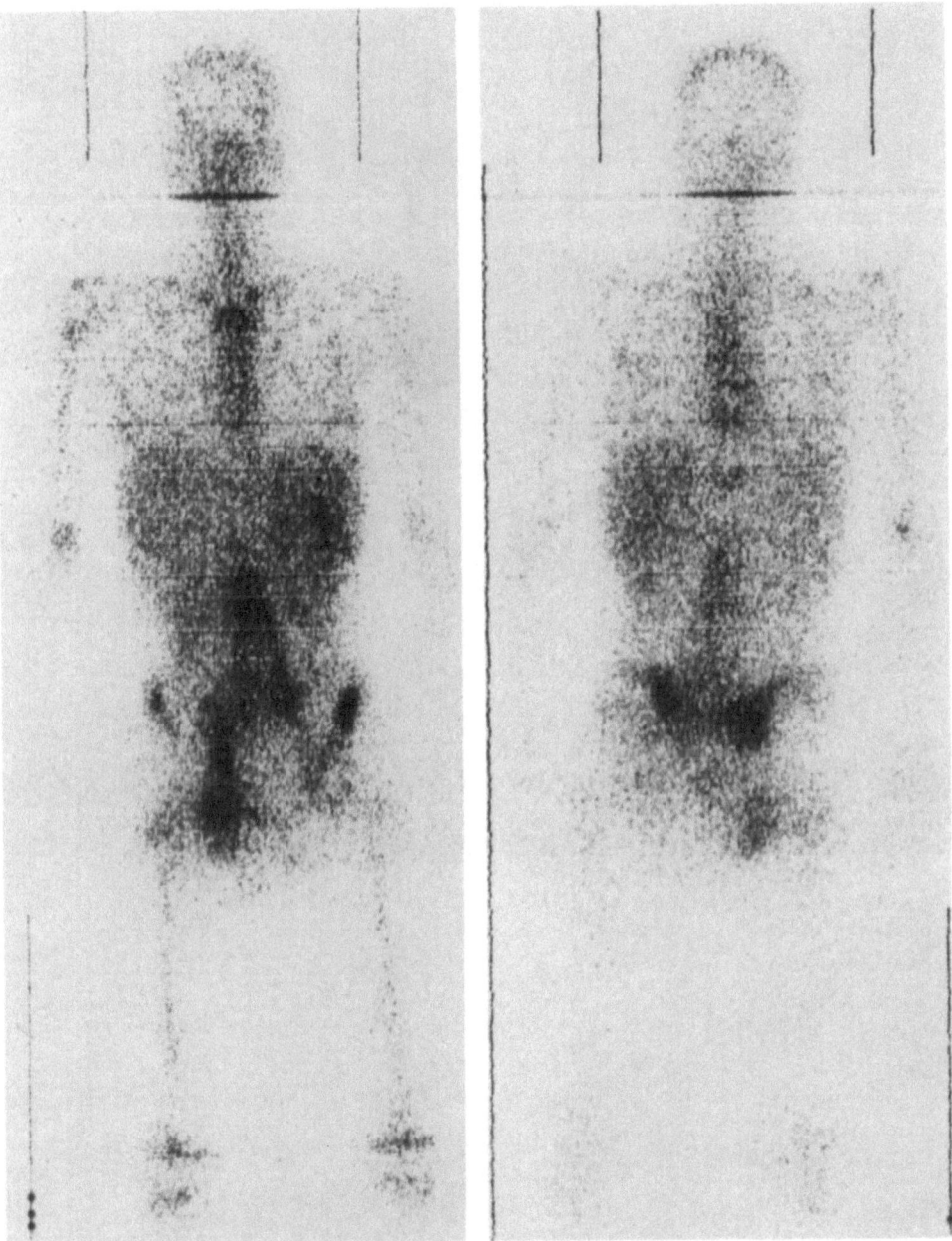

Fig. 7-11C. Hodgkin's disease - Sequential Studies (continued):
Eleven months after the preceeding study (Fig. 7-11B), while still
on therapy, right inguinal adenopathy developed. This 67-Ga scan
indicates extensive relapse involving the paraaortic, iliac and
right inguinal nodes and the right ischium. Bone x-rays and scans
also showed abnormalities in the right ischium.

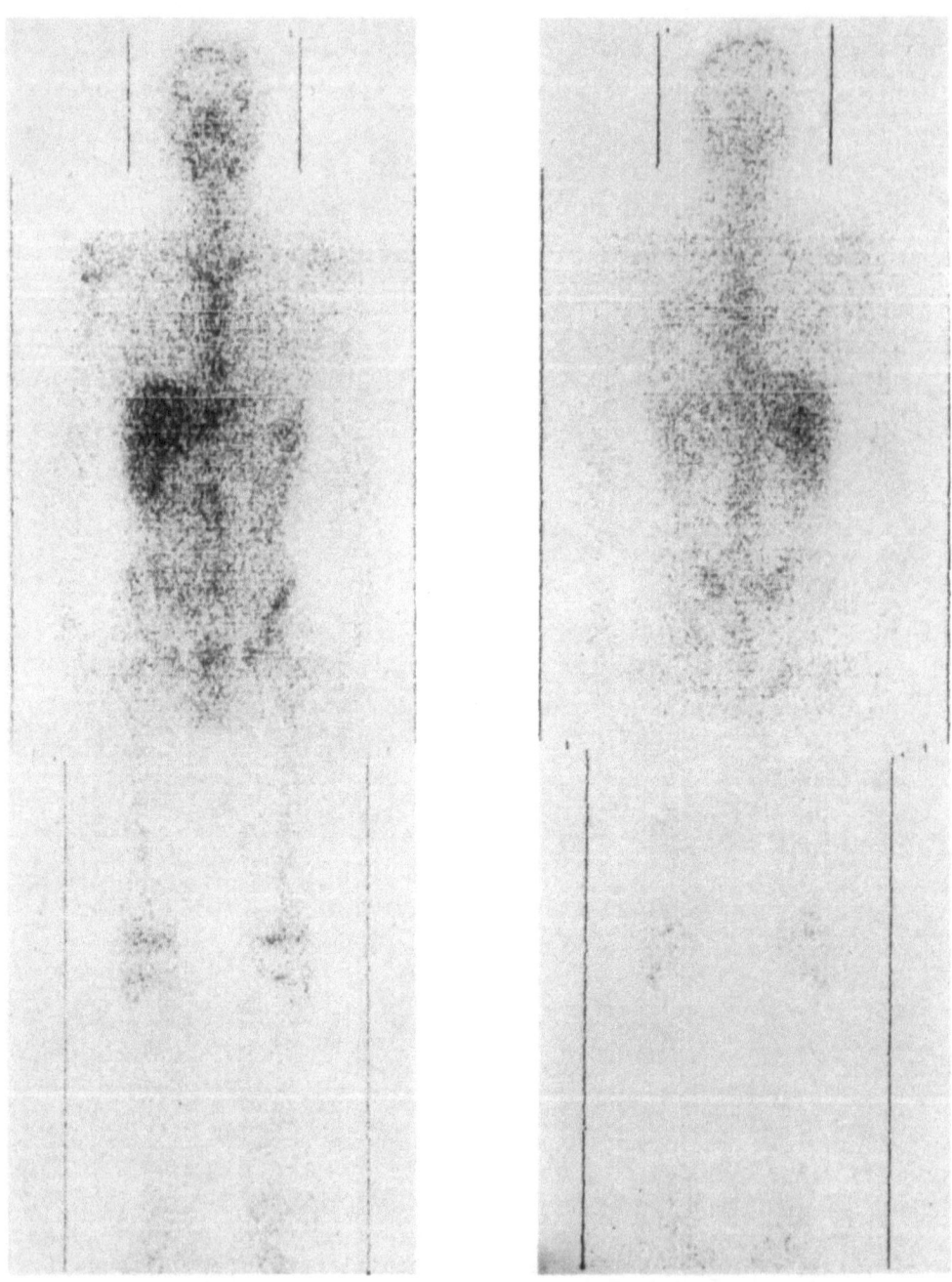

Fig. 7-11D. Hodgkin's disease – Sequential Studies (continued):
After three weeks of bleomycin, this 67-Ga scan suggests resolution
of all the previously seen tumor. This was confirmed by clinical
and radiological examination and he again was in complete remission.

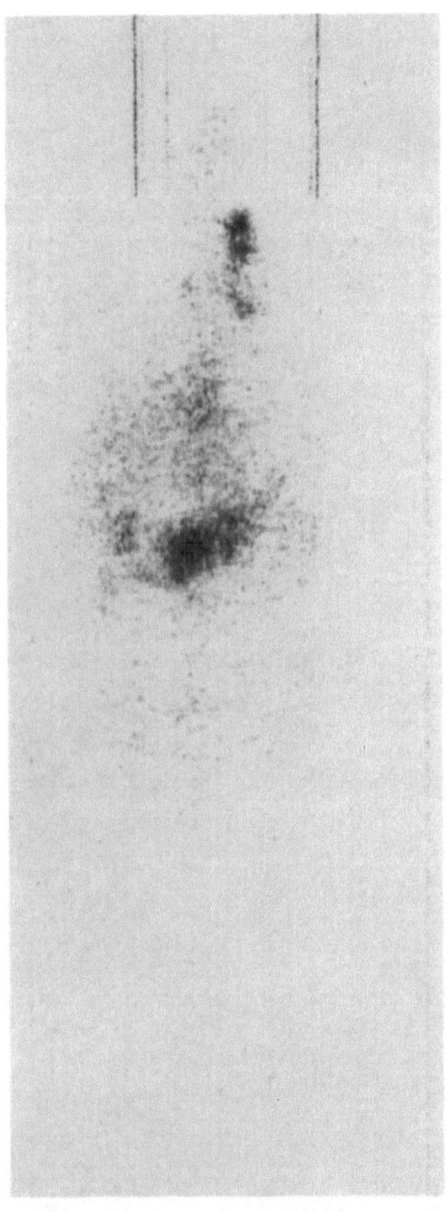

Fig. 7-12A. Malignant Lymphoma, lymphocytic, poorly differentiated –
Sequential Studies: First admission: A 54-year-old man developed
left cervical adenopathy which was biopsied and found to be lymphoma.
This was determined to be stage III because of mediastinal adenopathy
on chest x-ray and a positive lymphangiogram. This 67-Ga scan
confirms the presence of left cervical, mediastinal and paraaortic
lesions as well as bilateral supraclavicular uptake. Subsequent
to splenectomy, he was treated with combination chemotherapy.

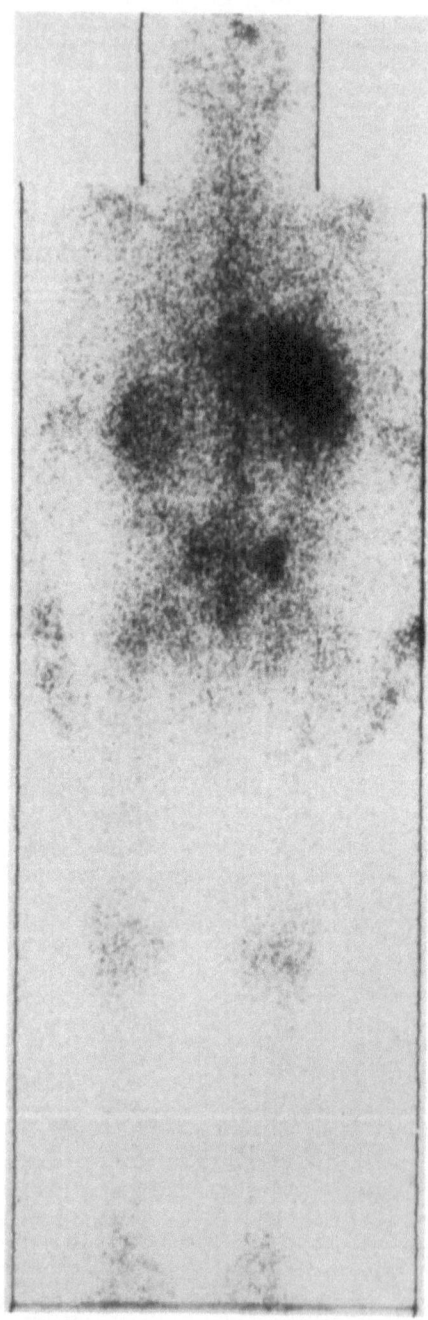

Fig. 7-12B. Second admission: Nine months later he developed
seizures and a brain scan was positive. This repeat 67-Ga study
shows a right brain mass and absence of all previous lesions.
The brain mass regressed after local radiotherapy.

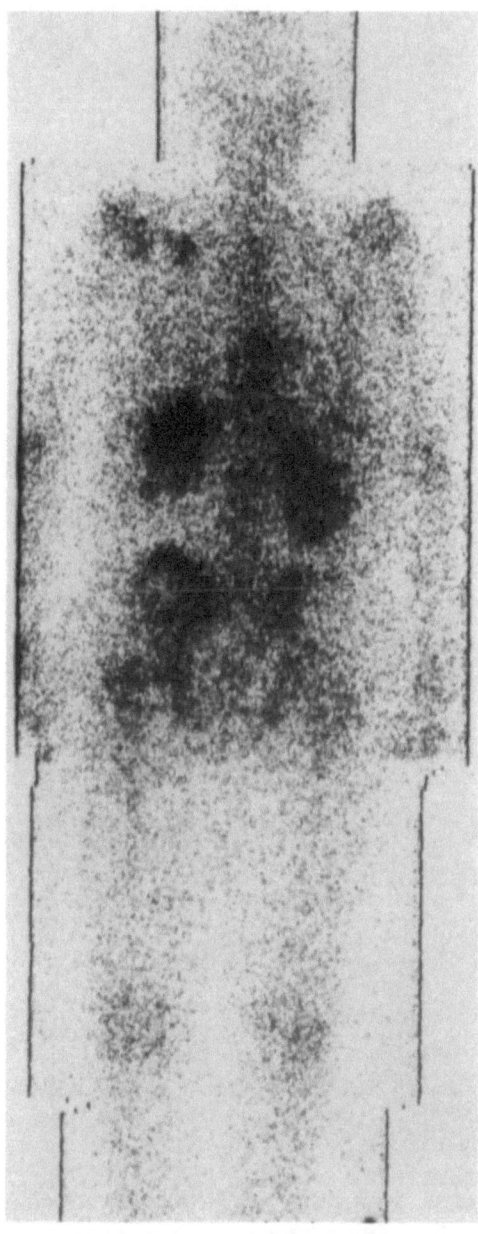

Fig. 7-12C. Third admission: Three months later he developed
widespread recurrence with hepatic failure and hematuria. An IVP
showed large kidneys. This 67-Ga scan shows a strikingly irregular
uptake in both kidneys and liver area and bony abnormalities in
the left shoulder, left hip and left iliac crest. At autopsy
shortly afterward, lymphoma was found involving the kidneys, liver,
bones, bladder, stomach and lymph nodes.

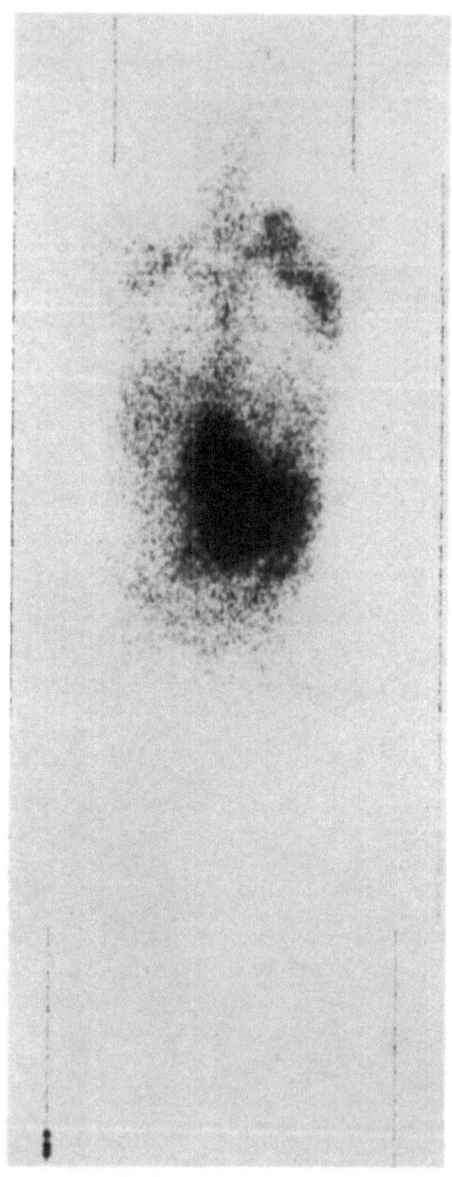

Fig. 7-13A. Malignant Lymphoma, histiocytic - Sequential Studies:
First admission: A 65-year-old man had a five-month history of
cervical adenopathy accompanied by fever, sweats, anorexia, and
weight loss. A biopsy showed lymphoma. Admission examination
showed axillary, supraclavicular and inguinal adenopathy. The
lymphangiogram was positive and the patient had marked thrombocytopenia. This anterior 67-Ga scan shows bilateral axillary,
left supraclavicular and massive abdominal involvement. Remission
was achieved with combination chemotherapy.

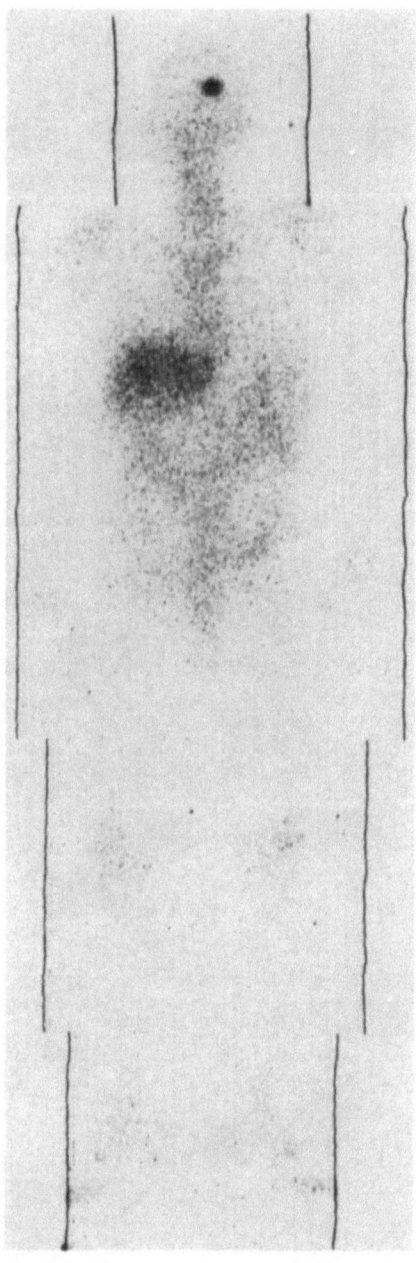

Fig. 7-13B. Second admission: Two years later the patient returned
with progressive gait disturbance, foot drop and disorientation.
This 67-Ga scan shows an intense area of uptake in the left frontal
region. A carotid arteriogram demonstrated a tumor in this region.
The patient was treated with local radiotherapy to the lesion
(Fig. 7-13C).

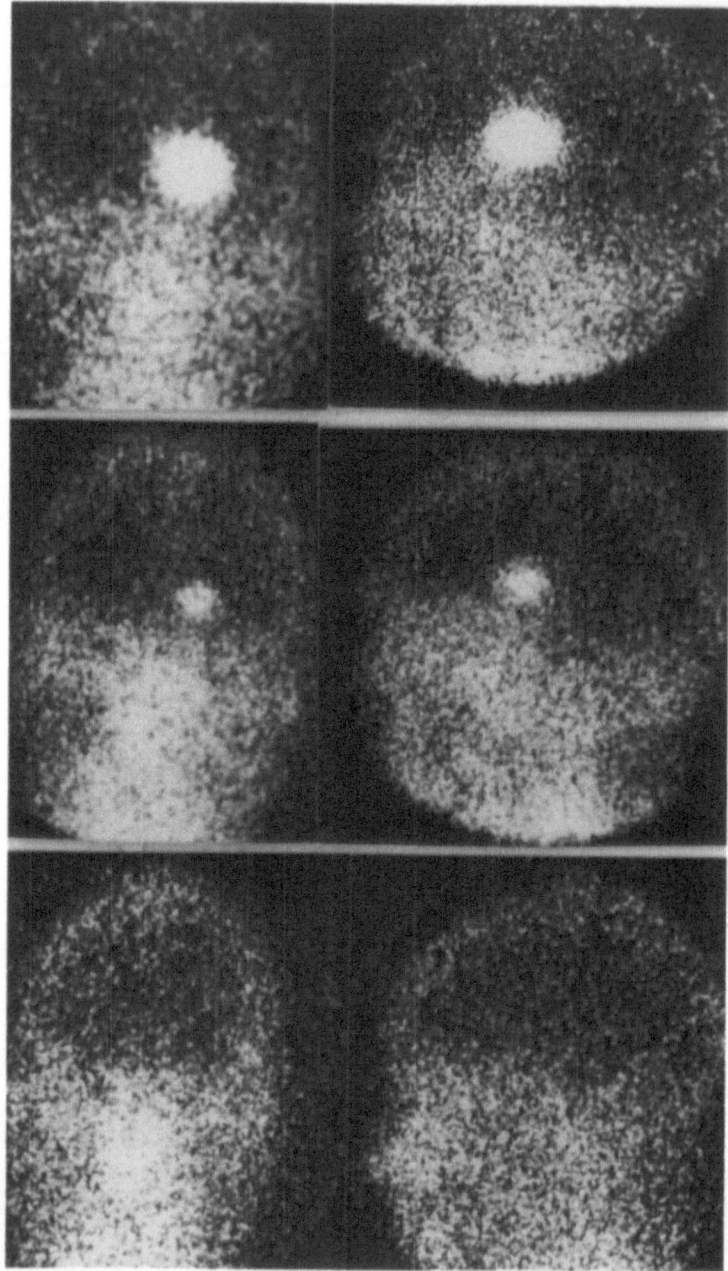

Fig. 7-13C. These serial 67-Ga brain scans document the disappearance of the mass seen on the anterior and left lateral views
on admission (top), after one week of radiotherapy (middle), and
after four weeks (bottom). The patient's cerebral symptoms cleared
concurrently. Refer to Fig. 11-10.

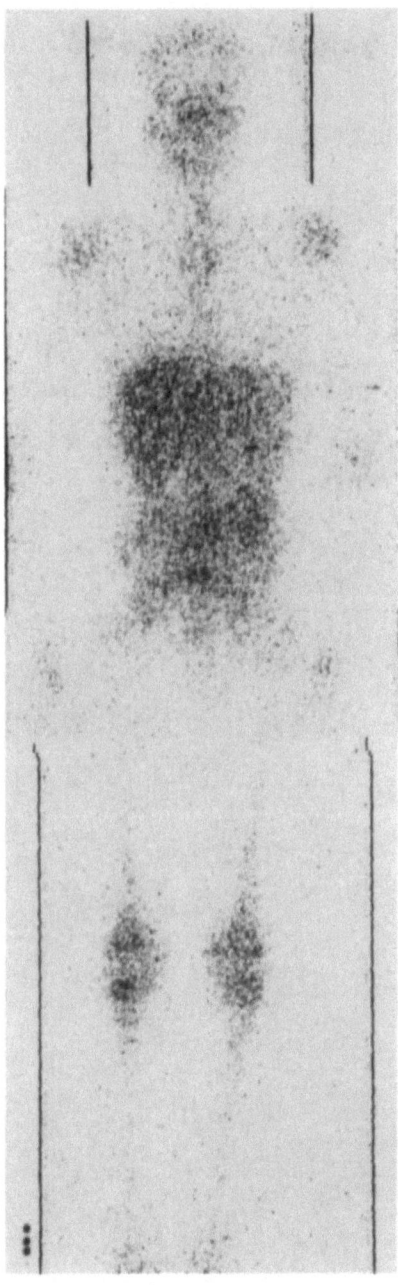

Fig. 7-14. Acute Myelocytic Leukemia: This 16-year-old male was found to have acute myelocytic leukemia with a bone marrow 85% replaced by myeloblasts. He was begun on chemotherapy. The anterior 67-Ga view reveals marked uptake throughout the long bones of the extremities with accentuation at the ends of the bones.

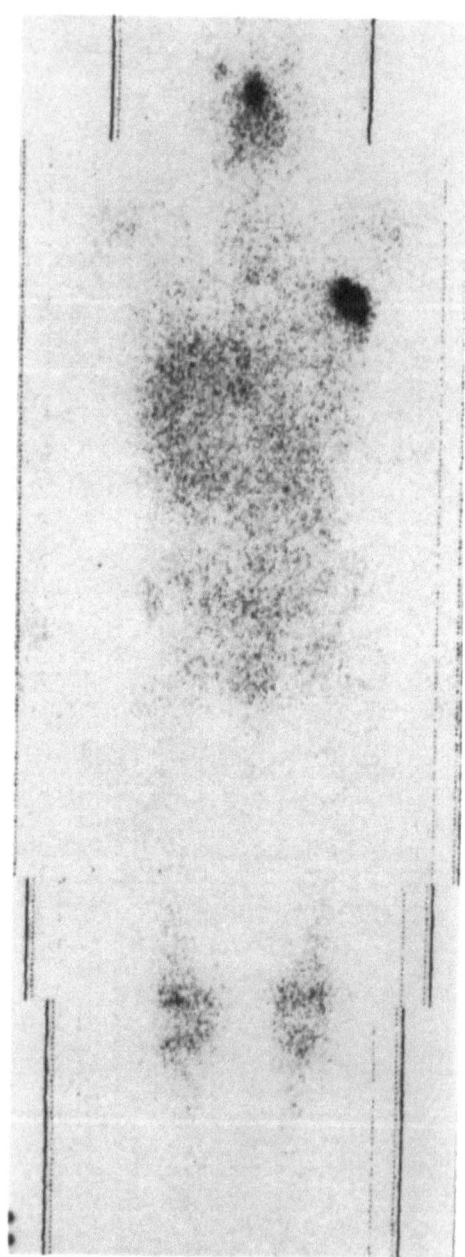

Fig. 7-15A. Acute Myeloblastic Leukemia - Myeloblastoma: A 15-
year-old girl presented with pallor, bleeding and a 5 cm left
breast mass. Her leukocyte count was 240,000 and her marrow
showed 90% myeloblasts. A nasopharyngeal mass was also found.
The anterior 67-Ga scan on admission shows 67-Ga concentration in
the left breast mass and prominent uptake in the nasal area.

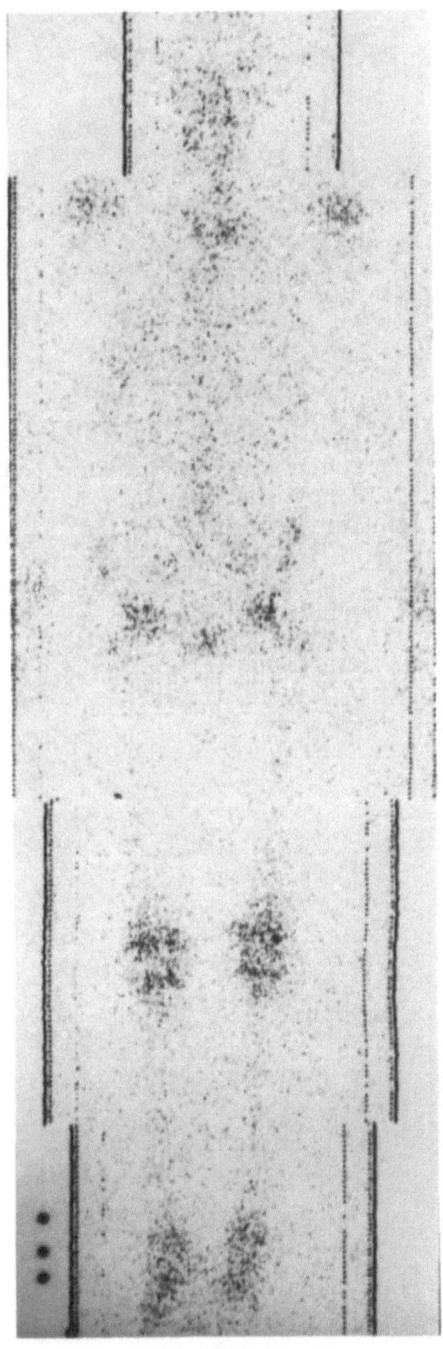

Fig. 7-15B. Acute Myeloblastic Leukemia - Myeloblastoma (continued):
After three weeks of treatment both masses had disappeared and the
67-Ga scan returned to normal.

Fig. 7-16. Acute Lymphocytic Leukemia:
A 15-year-old boy was found to have
acute lymphocytic leukemia with 95%
lymphoblasts in the bone marrow and
generalized adenopathy. His leukocyte
count was 10,000. This anterior 67-Ga
scan shows increased bone uptake in the
lower extremities and a large liver.
Lymph nodes are not visualized.

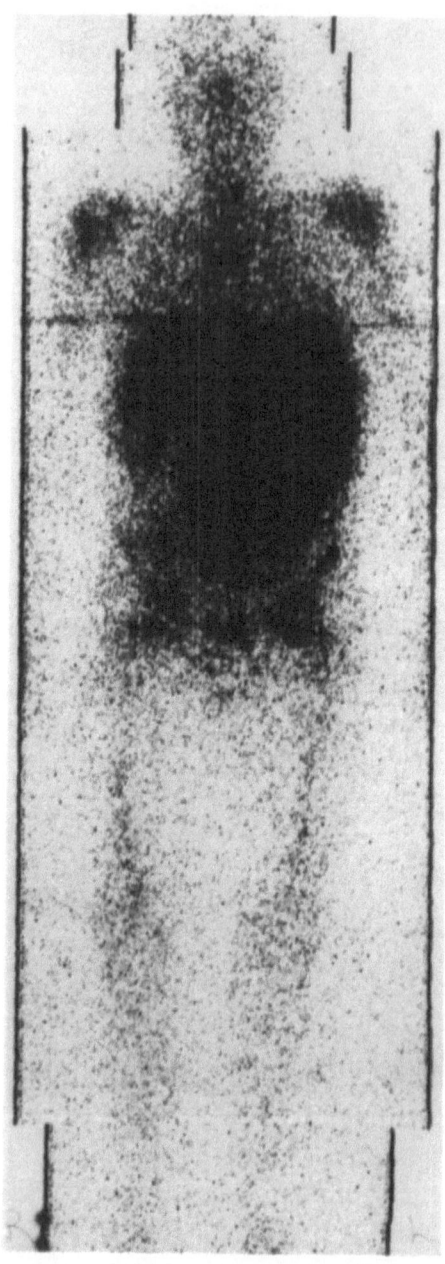

Fig. 7-17A.   Chronic Myelogenous Leukemia: First scan: A 37-year-old man developed anemia, weakness and a massively enlarged spleen. Bone marrow aspiration confirmed the diagnosis of CML.   The 67-Ga scan indicates intense uptake in the spleen which occupied most of the abdomen.   There was also increased concentration in the long bones of the lower extremities.

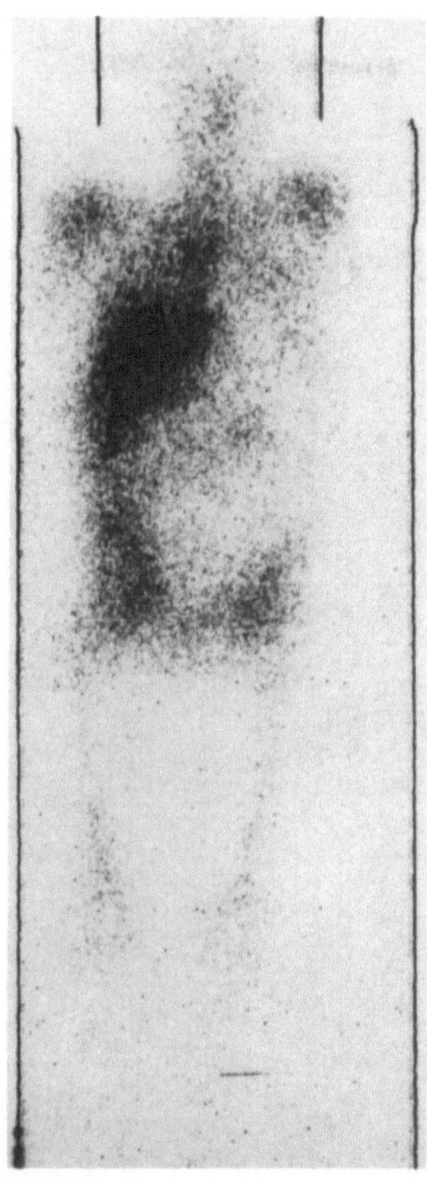

Fig. 7-17B. Chronic Myelogenous Leukemia (continued): Second
scan: Three weeks later he developed abdominal pain, jaundice,
nausea, and vomiting. A 99m-Tc sulfur colloid liver-spleen scan
showed no uptake in the spleen. This 67-Ga scan shows absent
uptake of 67-Ga where the large spleen had been observed on the
previous 67-Ga study. Follow-up: The patient died of sepsis
several days later. Autopsy revealed a complete septic infarction
of the spleen with thrombosis of the splenic artery and vein and
several other vessels.

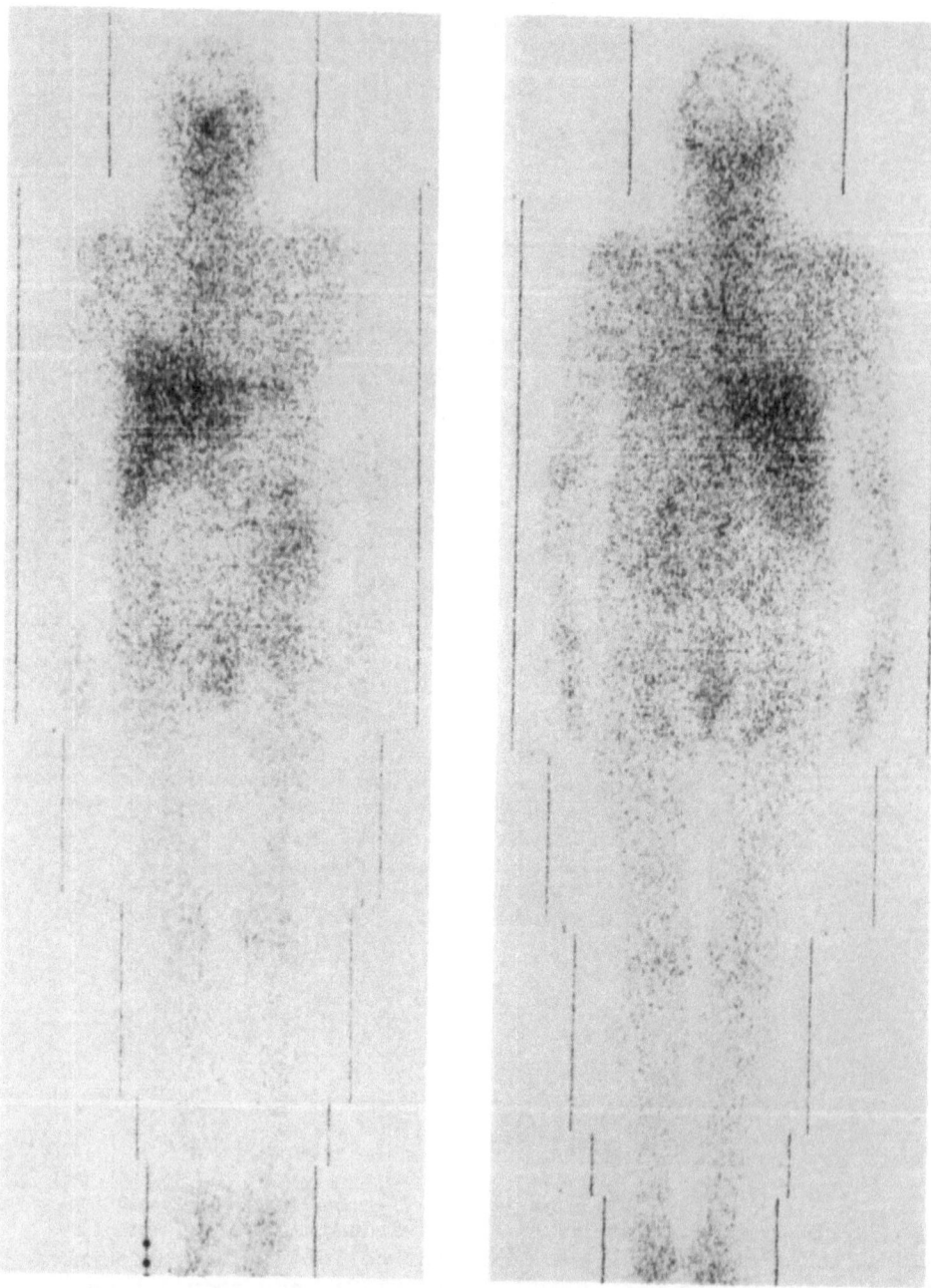

Fig. 7-18. Chronic Lymphocytic Leukemia: A 67-year-old woman
developed generalized adenopathy and anemia. The diagnosis of
CLL was made on findings in the peripheral blood, bone marrow
and lymph nodes. The 67-Ga scans show normal distribution of the
nuclide without any uptake in the diseased nodes or bone marrow.

CHAPTER 8

Gastrointestinal and Pelvic Tumors

Louis G. Gelrud, M. D. and Steven D. Richman, M. D.[*]

Section on Diseases of the Liver, Metabolic Diseases
    Branch, National Institute of Arthritis, Metabolism
    and Digestive Diseases

and

[*]Department of Nuclear Medicine, Clinical Center

National Institutes of Health, Bethesda, Maryland

Various malignancies of the abdomen and retroperitoneal areas
have been observed to accumulate the radionuclide 67-Ga (18,19,20,
24,29,36,54,55,56). Both primary and metastatic disease have been
visualized and the agent has been useful in delineating both carcinomas and lymphomas. The 67-Ga scintiscan has been helpful in
detecting unsuspected sites of neoplastic involvement and in
delineating the extent of neoplastic spread within a given area.
In patients with malignant lymphoma, the agent has been useful in
defining the degree of lymph node involvement since it tends to be
concentrated within disease-laden lymphatic tissue (51). Thus, it
has become a valuable adjunct in 'staging' the degree of neoplastic
spread in this type of malignancy (50).

67-Ga scintiscans cannot differentiate neoplasm from inflammation since both are represented as areas of increased localization,
but the radionuclide has been used to detect suspected inflammatory
lesions (20,24,27,36,68). The ability of this agent to detect an
area of inflammation is dependent on the activity of the inflammatory process within the lesion (28). An acute, active process is
more likely to exhibit concentration of the isotope than a more
chronic lesion, although these latter lesions may be visualized
if an adequate inflammatory response exists.

119

The use of the 67-Ga scintiscan (48-72 hours after intravenous injection), to detect areas of abnormality within the abdomen, is made difficult because the predominant mode of excretion of the radionuclide is fecal (17). The 67-Ga accumulates within the lumen of the gut and may be visualized on the scintiscan. In an effort to remove the 67-Ga from the bowel, cathartics are routinely administered prior to scanning. Despite these measures an area of the abdomen is frequently visualized which may represent either an abnormality or 67-Ga accumulation within the feces. This may be resolved by the readministration of cathartics and rescanning of the patient 12 to 24 hours later. If the questionable area of 67-Ga activity has moved along the bowel or disappeared then fecal contamination may be assumed. If the area of 67-Ga activity persists, even after catharsis and normal bowel function, then an area of abnormal pathology is suspected.

In summary, the excretion of 67-Ga into the GI tract with resulting fecal contamination may confuse interpretation of the scintiscan. This problem is circumvented when the bowel is adequately cleansed. In this situation, the 67-Ga scintiscan becomes useful in detecting neoplastic or inflammatory lesions of the GI tract.

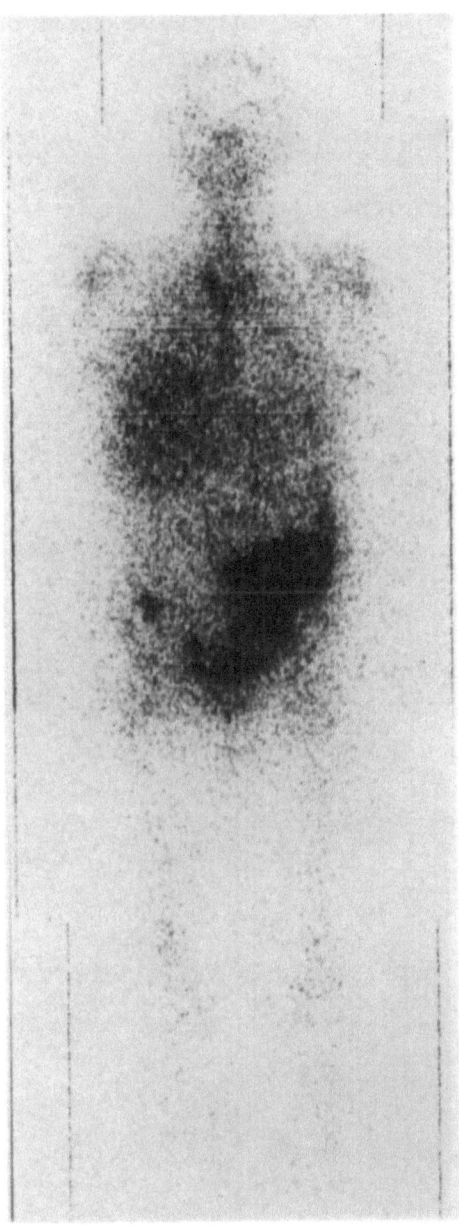

Fig. 8-1. A 42-year-old woman was found to have a pelvic mass on routine examination. She subsequently had an exploratory laparotomy with the biopsy diagnosis of cystadenocarcinoma of the ovary. This anterior 67-Ga scan demonstrates abnormal activity in the region of the left lower abdomen at the site of her tumor mass. There is also increased activity in the right lower abdomen representing metastatic disease.

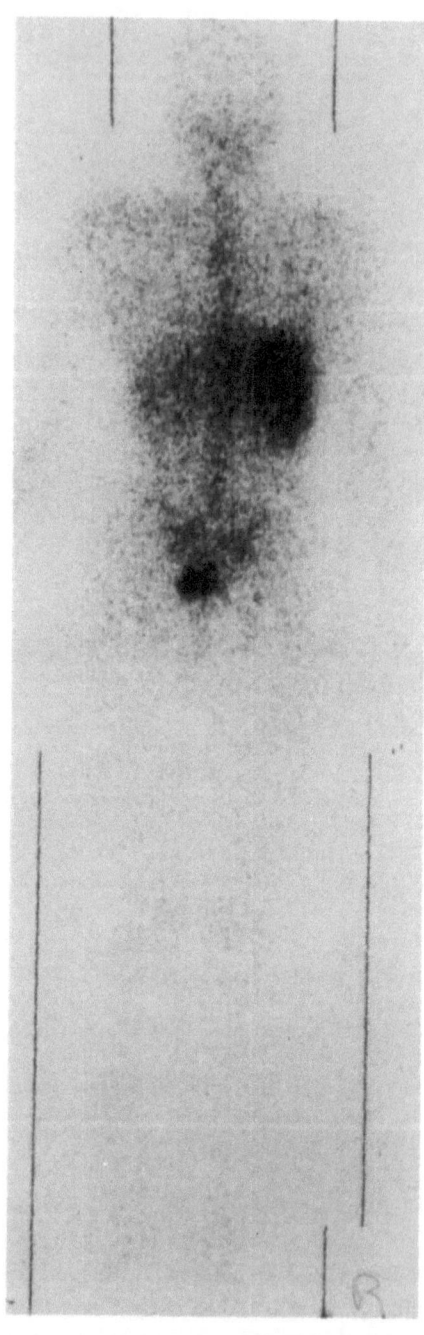

Fig. 8-2.   A 26-year-old woman entered with bleeding per vagina
secondary to recurrent carcinoma of the cervix.   The posterior
67-Ga scan demonstrates localized increase of activity in the
region of recurrent tumor of the cervix.

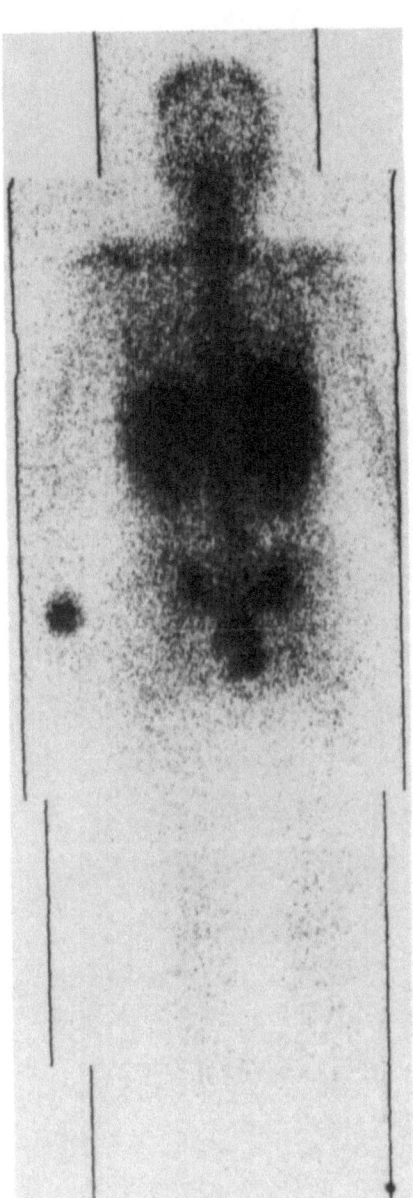 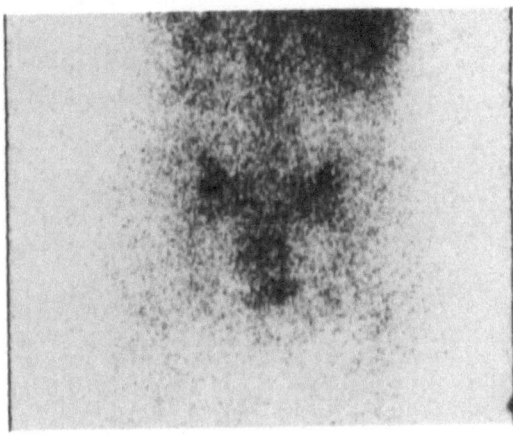

Fig. 8-3. A 55-year-old woman with history of abdominoperineal
resection for adenocarcinoma of the rectum was admitted with
recurrent tumor. Surgical exploration revealed an unresectable
mass in the mid-pelvis in the bed of the rectum. The posterior
67-Ga scan on the left, obtained prior to surgical exploration,
shows abnormal activity in the region of recurrent rectal tumor.
A repeat posterior 67-Ga scan two days after the first scan reveals
increased activity remaining in the pelvis.

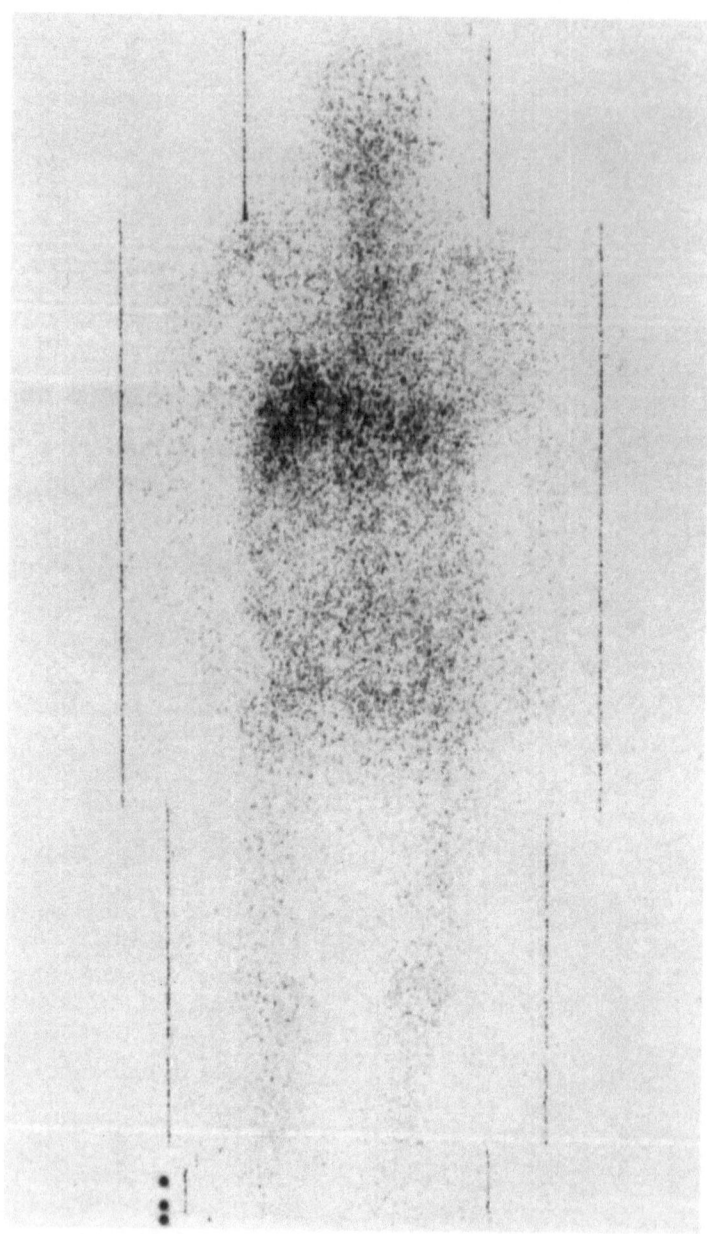

Fig. 8-4. A 54-year-old female was admitted with a one-year
history of diarrhea. A large vascular tumor of the head of the
pancreas was diagnosed by superior mesenteric arteriogram. Exploratory laparotomy revealed a surgically unresectable "delta cell"
tumor of the pancreas. This 67-Ga scintiscan shows an abnormal
accumulation of activity in the mid epigastric region corresponding to the site of the pancreatic tumor.

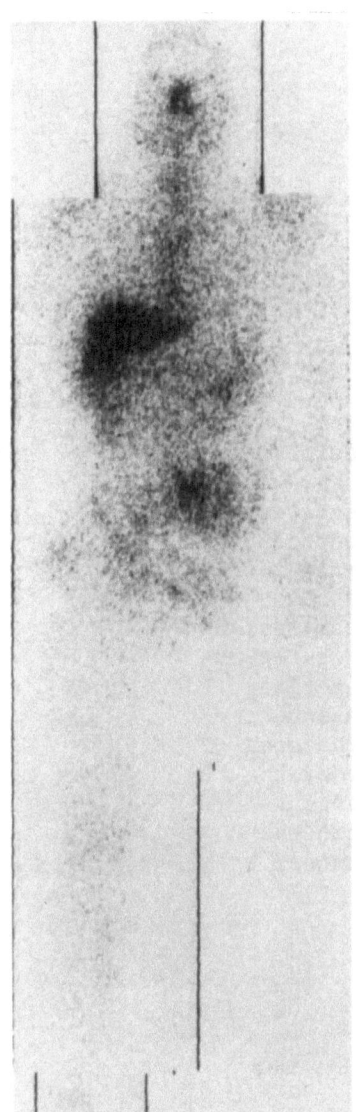 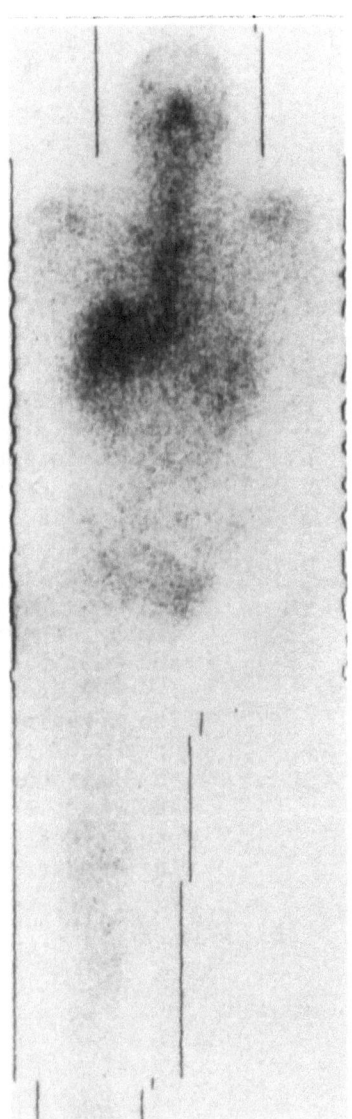

Fig. 8-5. A 33-year-old man was studied 3 years after a modified left hemipelvectomy for myxo-liposarcoma of the left posterior thigh. Bone scan with 99m-Tc polyphosphate demonstrated an abnormal accumulation in the right hip region. 67-Ga scan confirmed this finding and also showed accumulation of activity in the left pelvis. Abnormal neovascularity and tumor stain in the left pelvis was seen on mesenteric arteriogram. The anterior 67-Ga scan on the left shows activity in the right hip region and in the left pelvis. Following radiation therapy, the 67-Ga scan on the right demonstrates resolution of the abnormalities in the right hip and in the left pelvis.

Fig. 8-6. A 16-year-old boy with
Fanconi's anemia and acute granulocytic
leukemia developed Pseudomonas aeruginosa
septicemia. A Pseudomonas aeruginosa abscess was present in the left buttock.
Symptoms developed of disseminated intra-
vascular coagulopathy and bowel obstruc-
tion. At autopsy, a left buttock lesion
and multiple ulcerative lesions surrounding the ileocecal valve were described.
The anterior 67-Ga scan reveals intense
uptake of the radionuclide in the area of
the left buttock and right side of the
abdomen. Both areas were believed to represent 67-Ga accumulation within the
inflammatory lesions seen at autopsy.

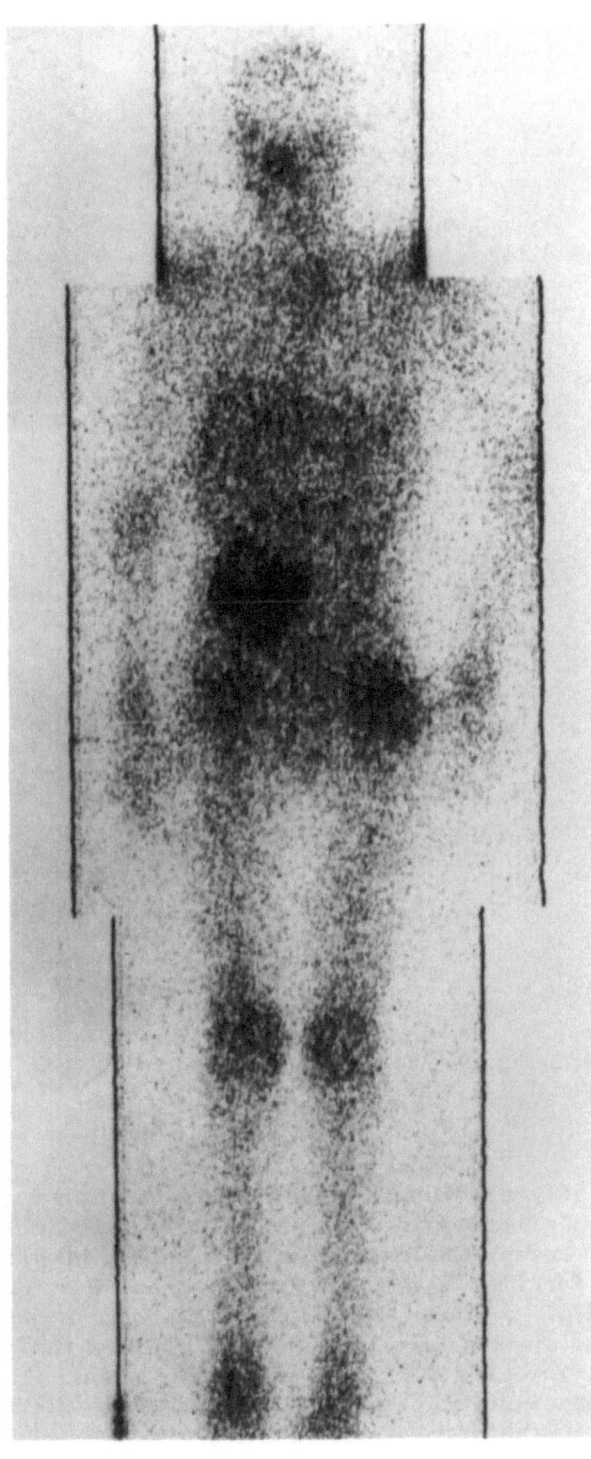

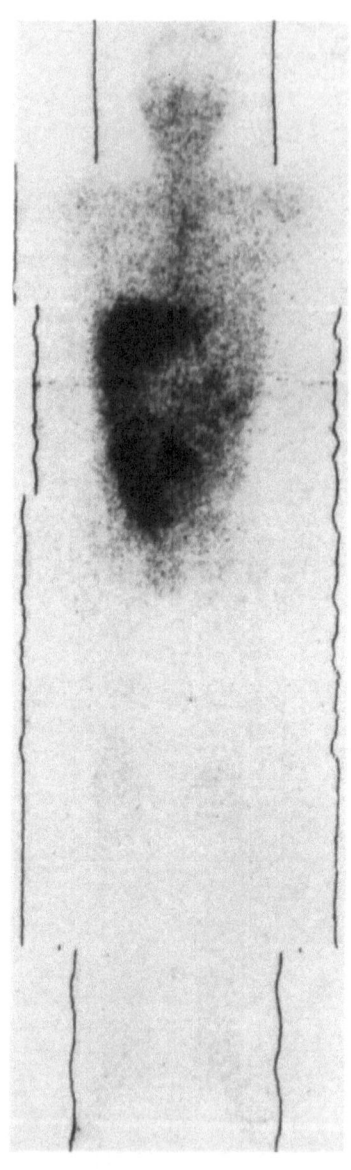 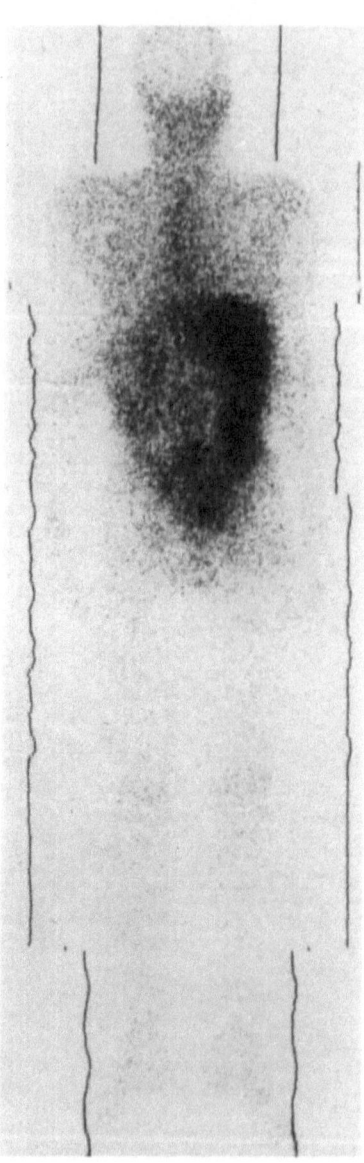

Fig. 8-7A. An 18-year-old man with a 3 years' history of metastatic pheochromocytoma of the spine, pelvis, femurs, and ribs was treated with radiation therapy and chemotherapy. Recent hepatomegaly without abnormal liver function studies was thought to be secondary to tumor involvement. A liver-spleen scan was interpreted as normal. The 67-Ga scans show an enlarged liver with increased radionuclide accumulation in the inferior portion of the right lobe. Three suspicious areas of increased uptake, believed to represent additional tumor metastases, were found in the upper and lower mid-abdomen and in the right inferior pelvis.

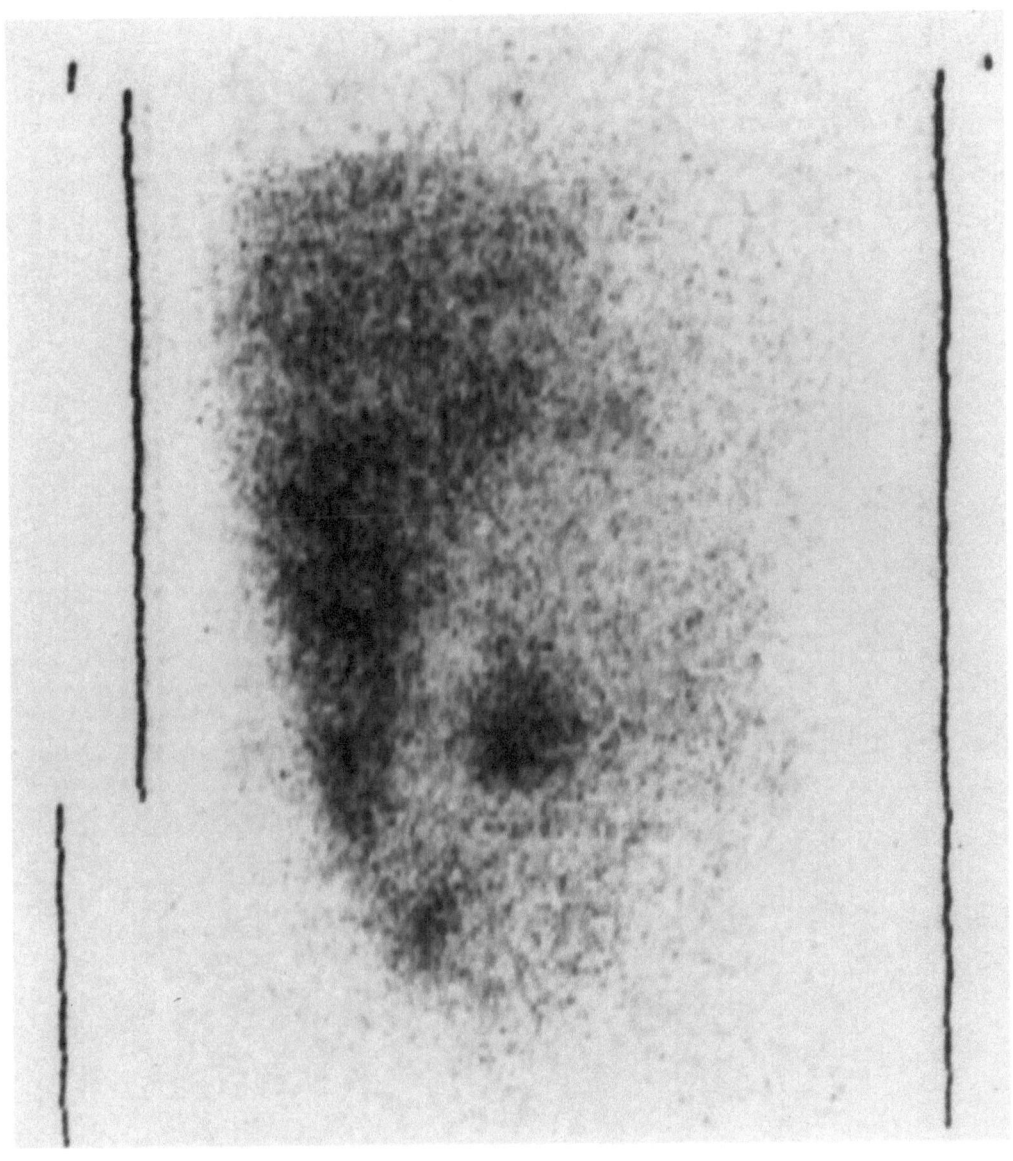

Fig. 8-7B. Repeat scan of the abdomen 20 hours later following catharsis showed no change in these sites of 67-Ga localization, thereby increasing the conviction that they represented sites of metastasis.

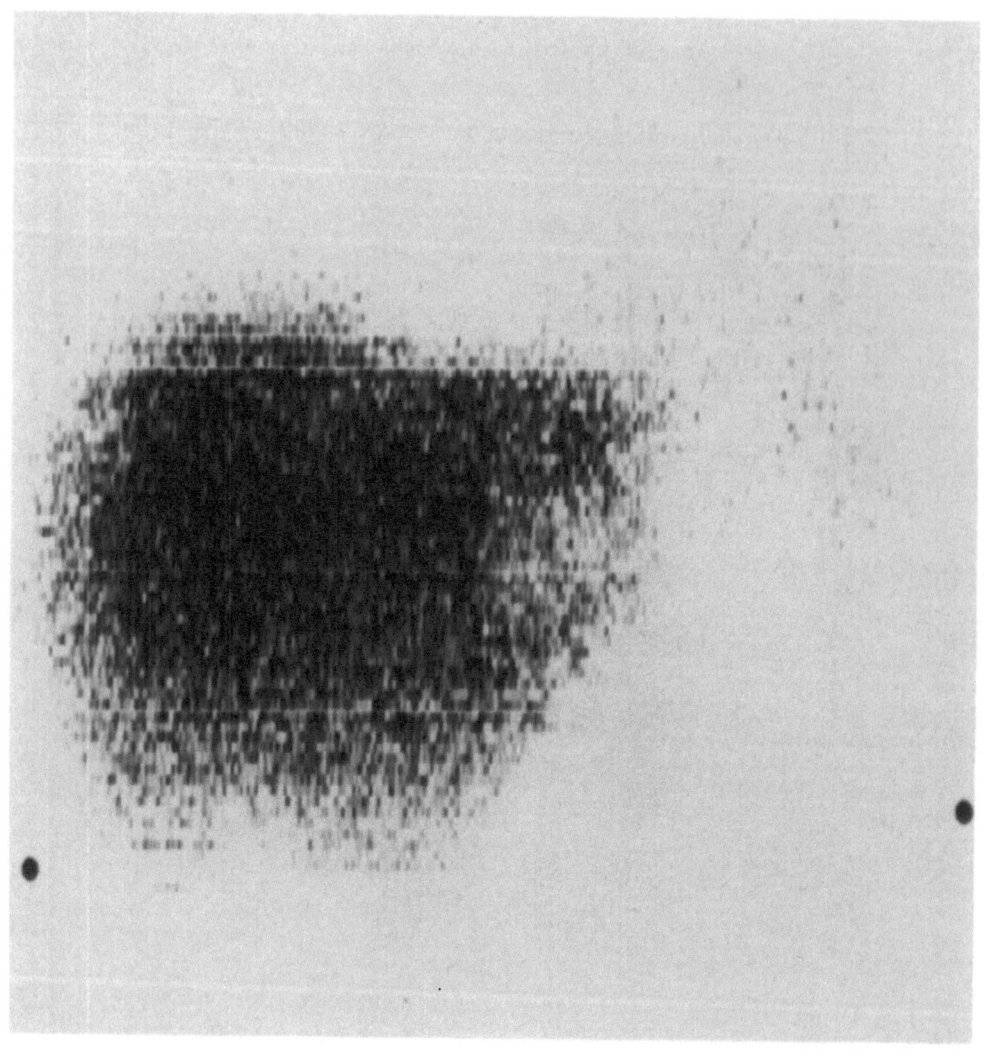

Fig. 8-8A. A 63-year-old woman with metastatic breast carcinoma
was seen at peritoneoscopy to have an enlarged left lobe of the
liver with gross metastases. Liver biopsy confirmed the presence
of metastatic disease. This anterior liver scan with 99m-Tc sulfur
colloid demonstrates a discrete defect in the left lobe of the liver.

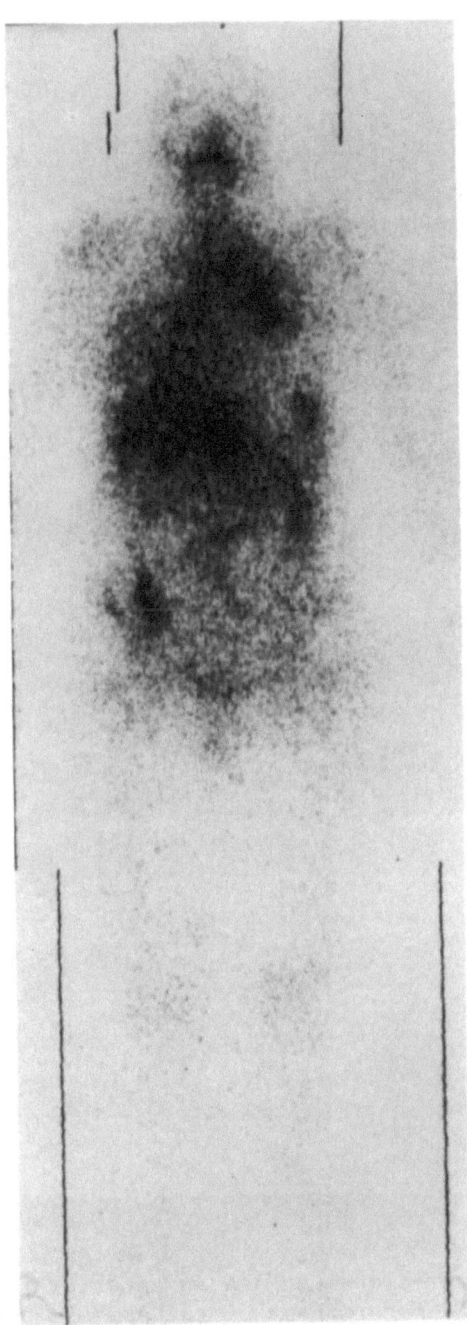

Fig. 8-8B. This anterior 67-Ga scan shows increased 67-Ga uptake
in the region of the metastatic focus in the liver (Compare with
Fig. 8-8A). In addition, 67-Ga accumulation is present in the
pelvic bones, the ribs and in the left lung.

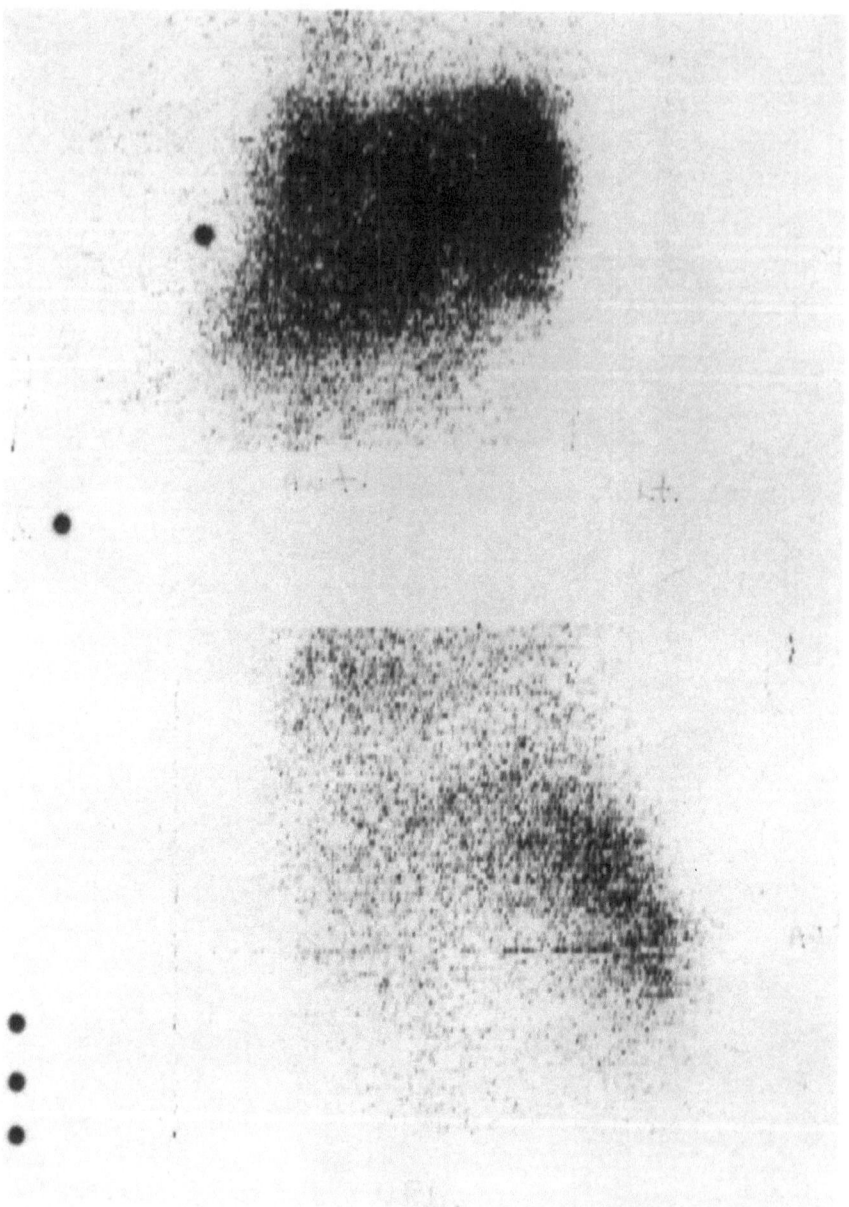

Fig. 8-9A. A 49-year-old woman had an anterior resection of a
large obstructing adenocarcinoma of the sigmoid one year before
this admission. Ascites and jaundice began two months prior to
this admission followed by progressive deterioration to hepatic
coma and death. Autopsy revealed diffuse metastatic adenocarcinoma.
The anterior liver scan with 99m-Tc sulfur colloid demonstrates a
large area of diminished uptake in the right lobe of the liver.

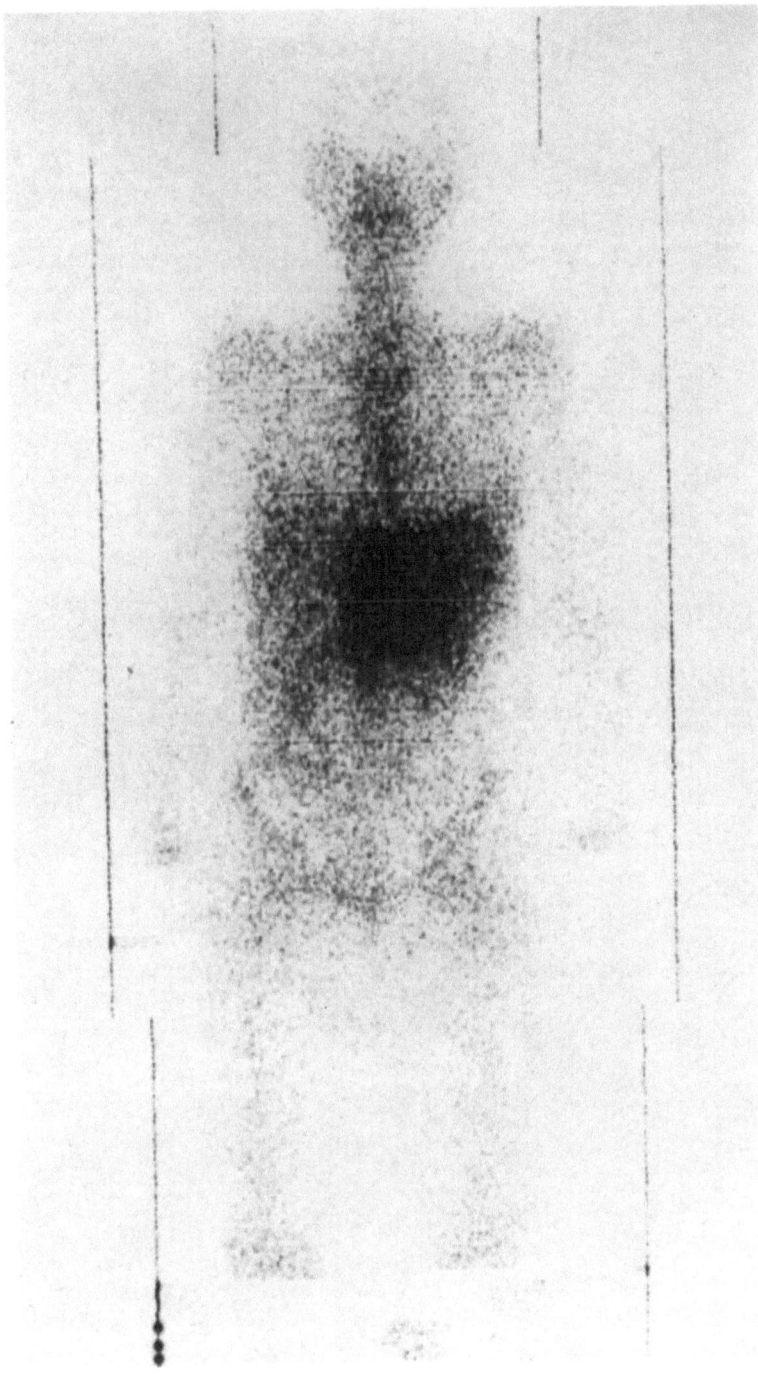

Fig. 8-9B. The anterior 67-Ga scan also demonstrates decreased activity throughout the right lobe.

CHAPTER 9

Breast Carcinoma

Robert S. Frankel, M. D. and Alfred E. Jones, M. D.

Department of Nuclear Medicine, Clinical Center

National Institutes of Health, Bethesda, Maryland

Breast carcinomas have been studied by several authors for their affinity for 67-Ga. Most studies show a less than 50% detection rate for adenocarcinomas of the breast. Our experience to date with this disease has been even less encouraging as far as detection of the primary lesions is concerned. In addition, normal breasts have, on occasion, been shown to accumulate 67-Ga. Therefore, differentiation of normal breast uptake from that in a breast carcinoma is difficult.

67-Ga scintigraphy, however, has been shown to be of considerable value in detecting the metastases of breast carcinoma. These include metastatic lesions to the skeletal system, brain, lungs, and other less commonly seen areas.

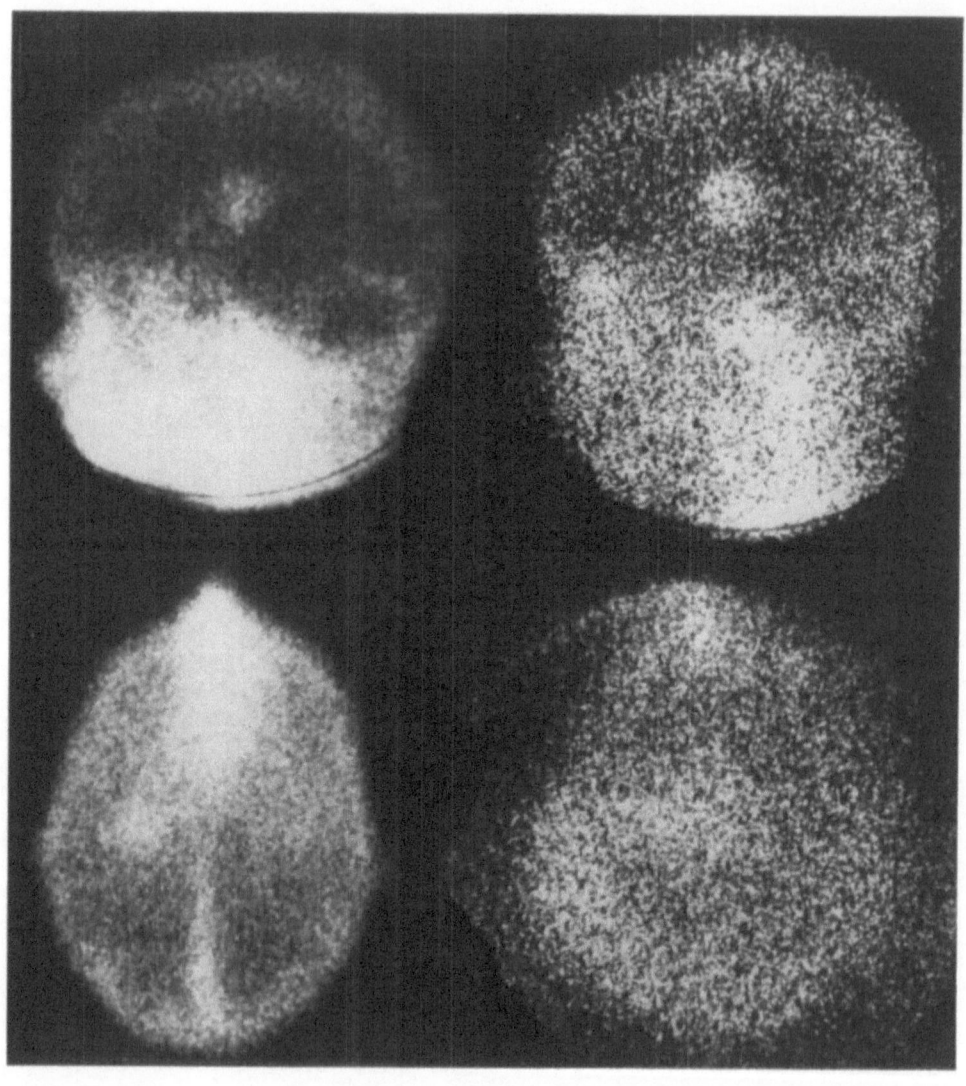

Fig. 9-1. 99m-Tc pertechnetate (left) and 67-Ga (right) brain
scans of a middle-aged woman with metastatic breast carcinoma.
Top row: left lateral views. Bottom row: vertex views. An area
of increased nuclide accumulation is seen in the left parietal
area on both studies. This proved to be a focus of metastatic
breast carcinoma at autopsy. This case illustrates the usefulness
of the gamma camera for 67-Ga imaging of the brain when looking
for metastases.

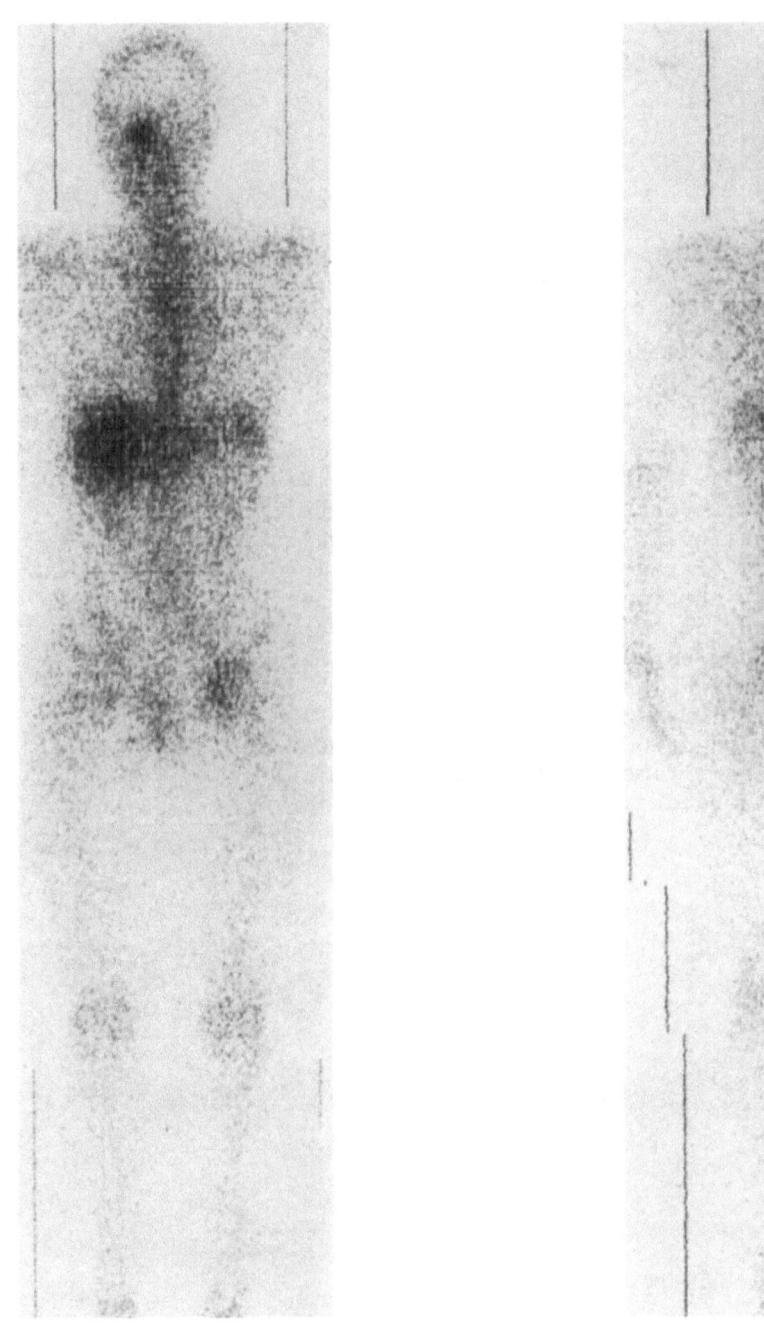

Fig. 9-2. 67-Ga scans of a patient with breast carcinoma meta-
tastic to bone. There are areas of increased accumulation in the
left sacro-iliac joint and left ischium. Neither of these areas
was depicted on x-ray at the time of this study.

Fig. 9-3. Thirty-year-old woman with
breast carcinoma metastatic to the liver.
Anterior 67-Ga scan shows massive enlarge-
ment of the liver with the left lobe oc-
cupying almost the entire left upper
quadrant of the abdomen. There are areas
of decreased 67-Ga accumulation seen in
the right hepatic lobe as well as in the
inferior edge of the left lobe. The areas
of absent 67-Ga uptake corresponded to
areas of absent uptake of 99m-Tc sulfur
colloid on a liver scan.

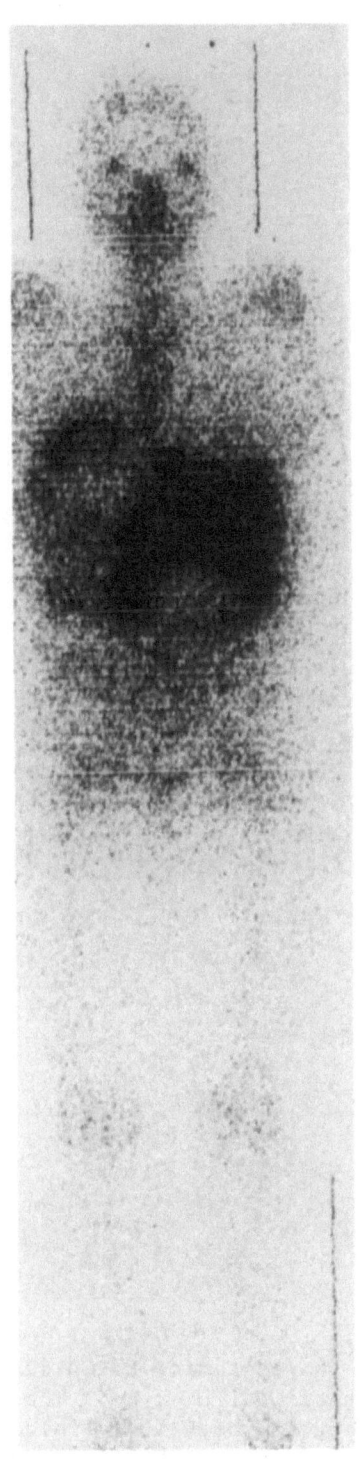

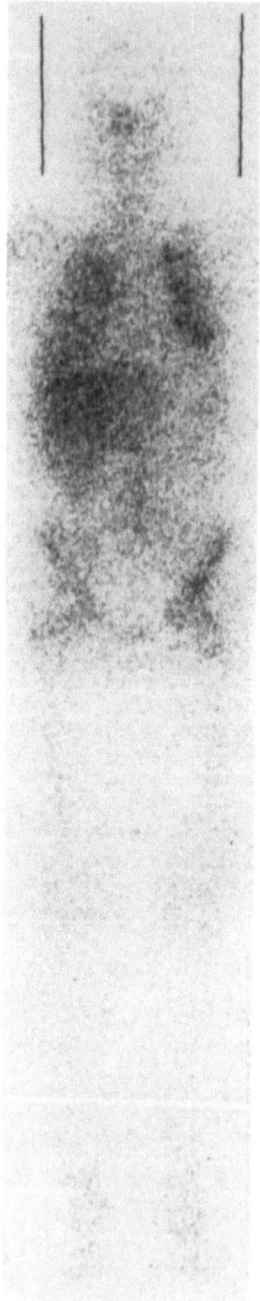 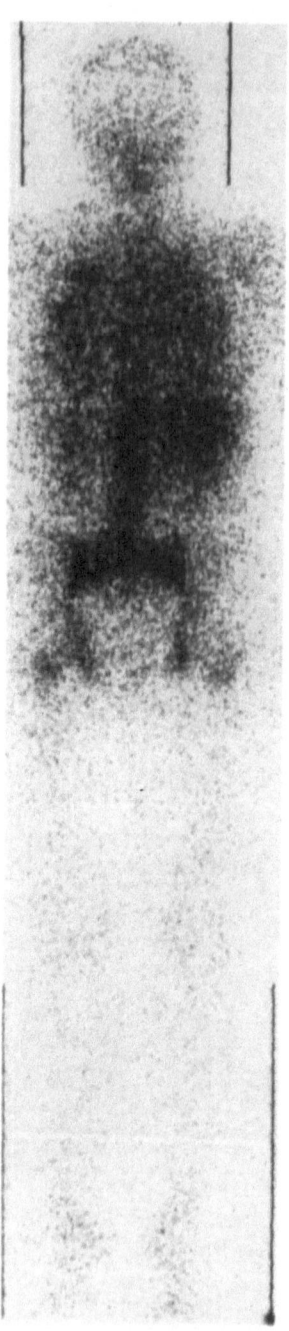

Figure 9-4A.   Anterior and posterior 67-Ga scans of a patient with breast carcinoma metastatic to the lung.   The scans show abnormal 67-Ga accumulation throughout both lung fields.   A PA chest x-ray (Fig. 9-4B) also shows diffuse metastatic disease bilaterally.

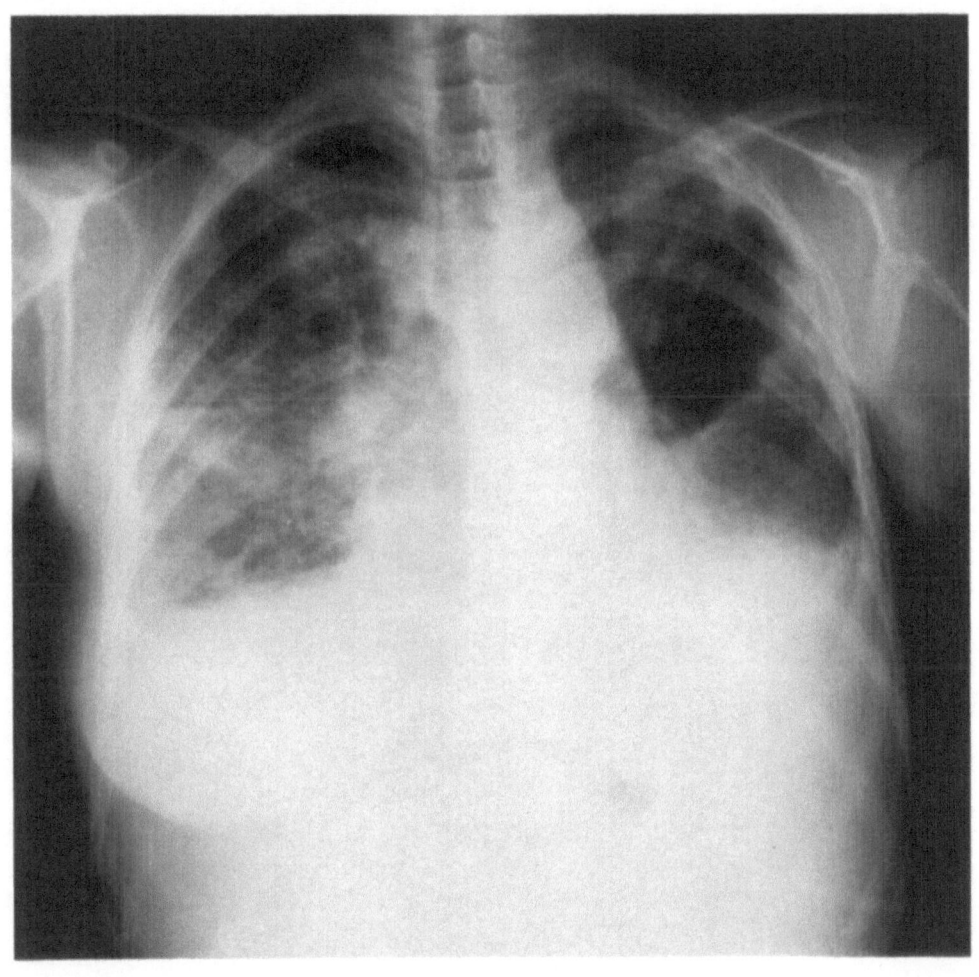

Fig. 9-4B

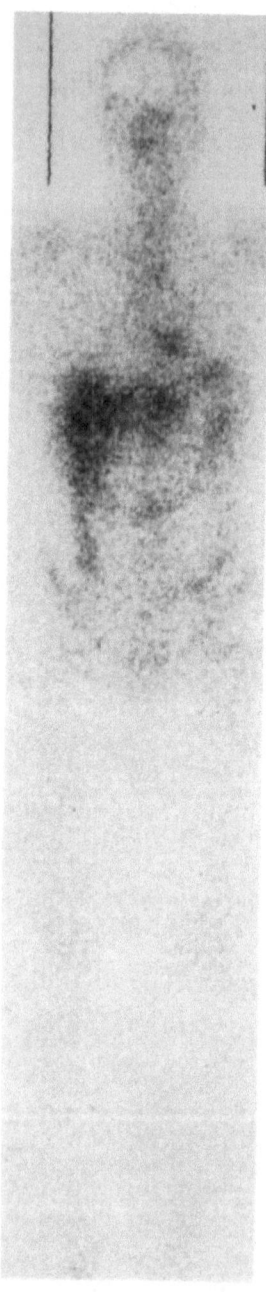

Fig. 9-5. Anterior whole body 67-Ga scan of a patient with cysto-
sarcoma phylloides involving the medial aspect of the left breast.
The tumor is visualized as an area of abnormal nuclide accumulation in the lower left chest region medially. The large bowel
is also seen as a normal variant.

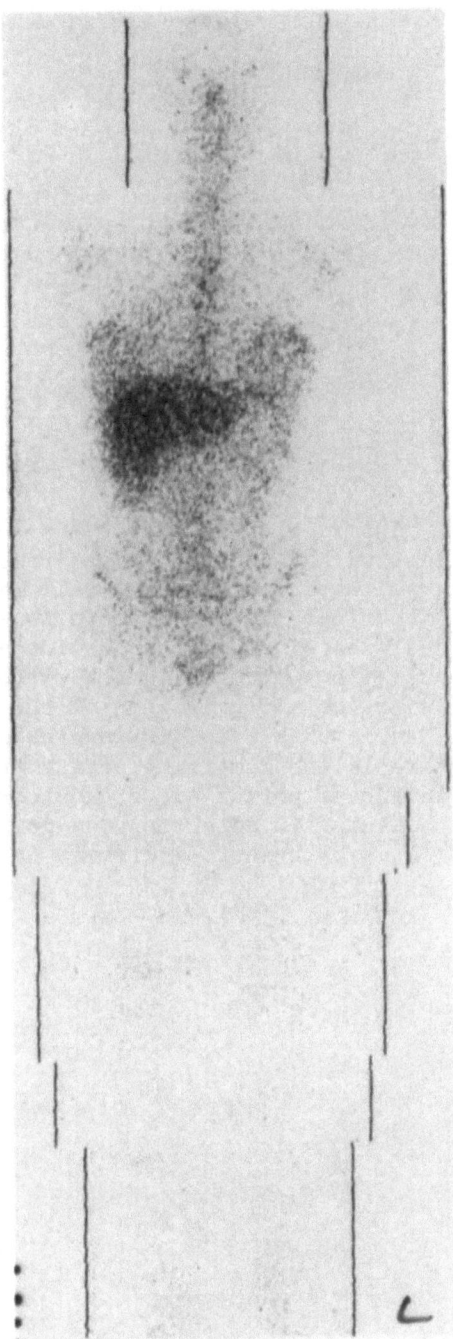

Fig. 9-6. Anterior whole body 67-Ga scan showing accumulation of radionuclide in the region of the breasts bilaterally. The patient had no evidence of breast disease.

Fig. 9-7. Anterior whole body 67-Ga scan
of a patient with a previous right radical
mastectomy with suspected chest wall recurrence on the right side. The scan shows an
ill-defined area of increased nuclide accumulation (arrow) in the right hemithorax
as well as uptake in the region of the left
breast. One is unable to distinguish physiologic uptake in the remaining breast from
tumor. This case points out a shortcoming
of 67-Ga scanning in detecting the primary
tumor in cases of breast carcinoma.

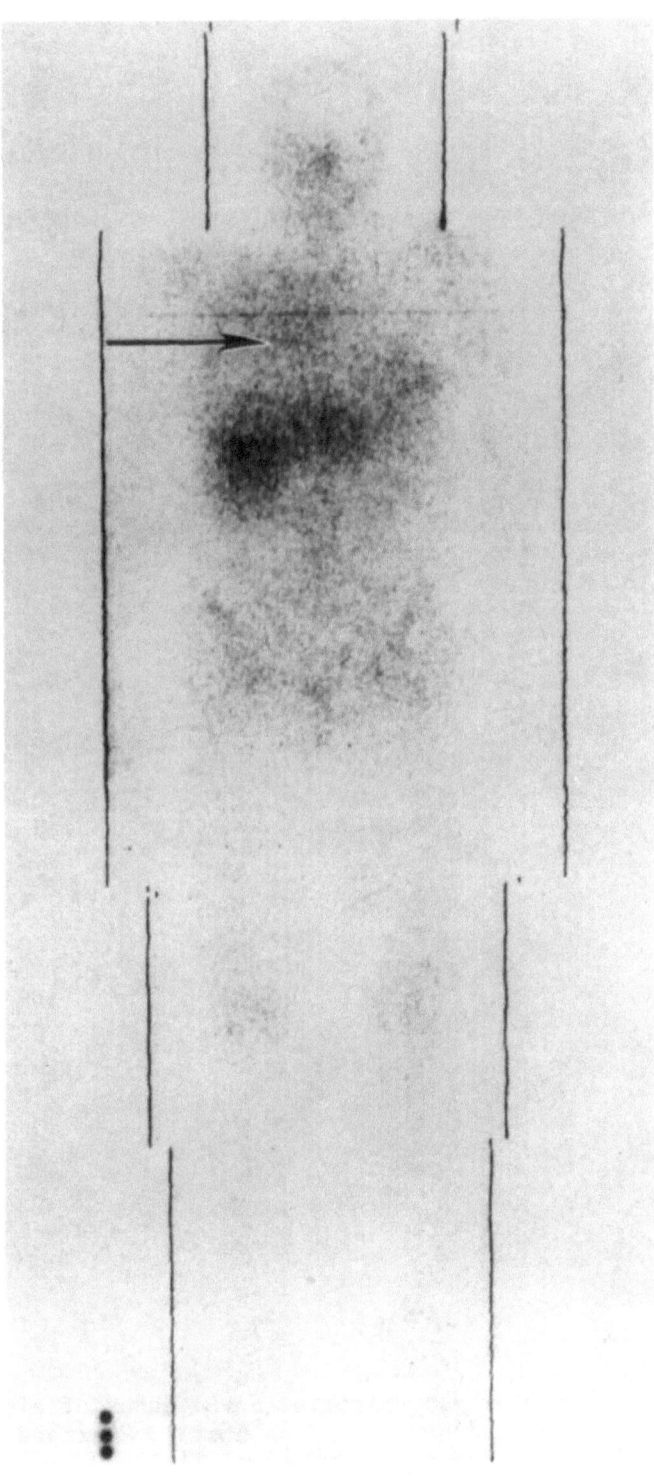

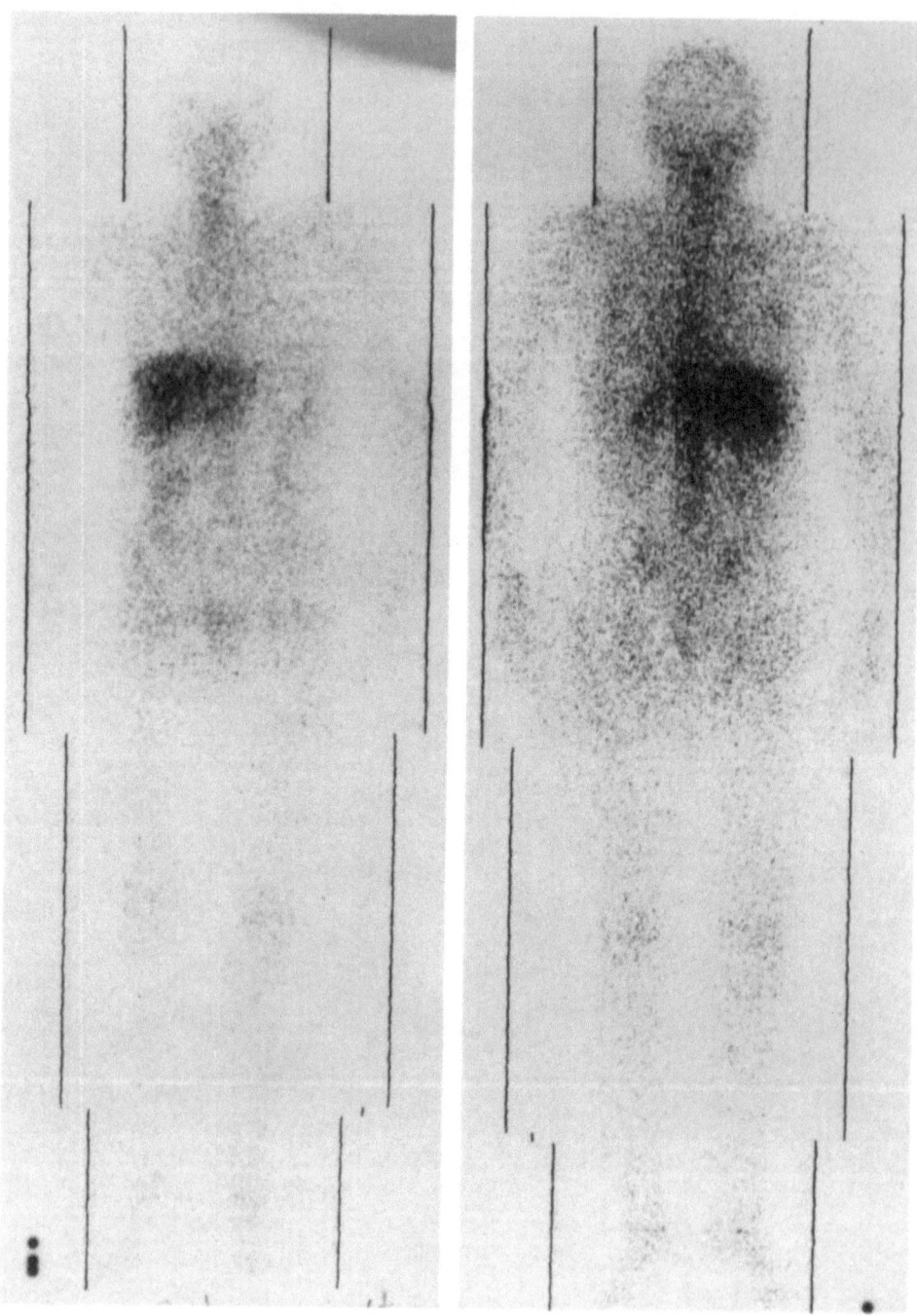

Fig. 9-8A. Anterior and posterior 67-Ga scans of a patient with adenocarcinoma of the breast and suspected metastases. The study was interpreted as being within normal limits.

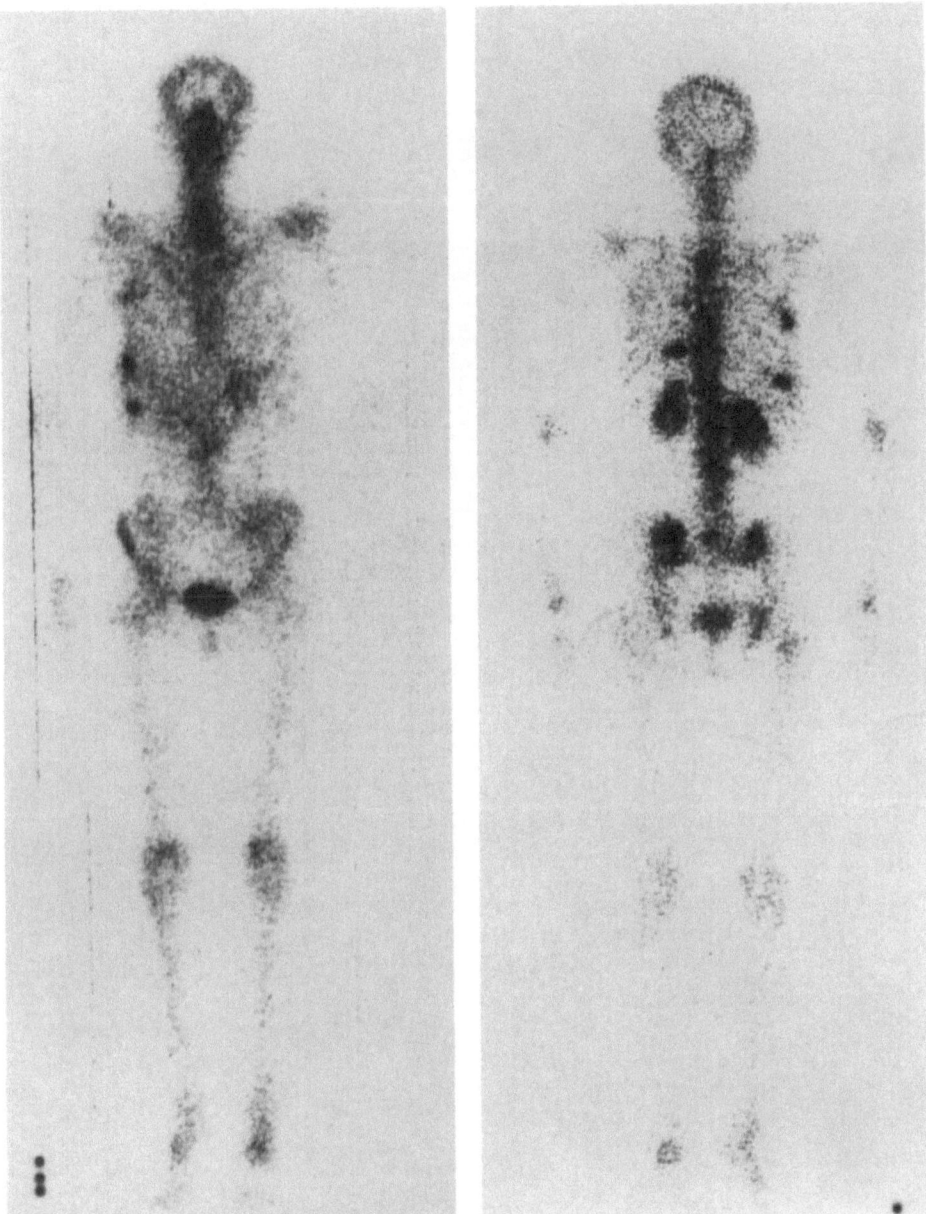

Fig. 9-8B. Anterior and posterior skeletal scans in the same
patient (Fig. 9-8A). Scanning was performed with 99m-Tc polyphosphate. Multiple rib lesions are evident. There is also
increased nuclide localization in the region of the lumbo-sacral
spine and the left sacro-iliac region. This comparison of scans
illustrates the frequent superiority of bone scans over 67-Ga
scans in skeletal metastases.

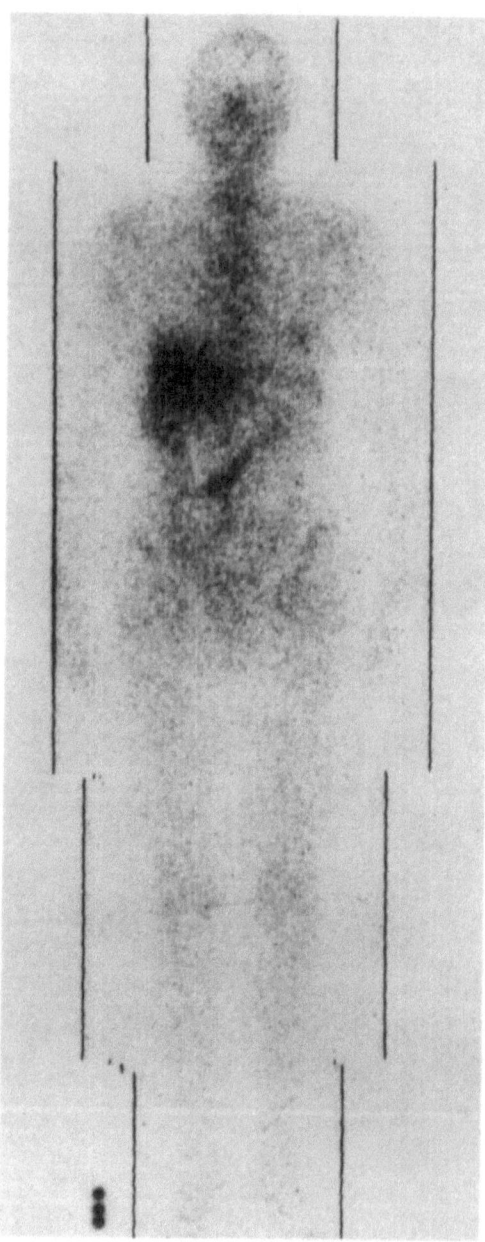

Fig. 9-9. Anterior whole body 67-Ga scan of a 47-year-old woman
showing increased 67-Ga accumulation in the region of the left
breast. No similar activity is seen in the region of the right
breast. The right breast was normal by clinical examination and
mammography. The area of 67-Ga localization in the left breast
was found to be carcinoma.

CHAPTER 10

Malignant Melanoma

Michael S. Milder, M. D.

Department of Nuclear Medicine, Clinical Center

National Institutes of Health, Bethesda, Maryland

Malignant melanoma is an uncommon tumor, accounting for about
1% of all cancers. However, it causes about as many deaths as the
more common cutaneous cancers (57). This tumor strikes adults of
all ages and metastasizes widely and unpredictably. Radical surgery
of localized lesions may provide five-year survival rates of better
than 50% with distant spread (58). Moreover, the tumor may recur
many years after treatment, so that long-term follow-up is necessary.
Survival has not been increased by radiotherapy, chemotherapy or
immunotherapy.

For all these reasons, detection of and surveillance for
metastatic spread are vitally important in the management and
counseling of the patient with malignant melanoma. Radioisotopic
methods for melanoma detection have been used previously. A 32-P
uptake test has been described for ocular melanomas (59). In
addition, an 125-I labelled chloroquine analogue that binds
specifically to melanin and differentiates melanoma from other
masses has been used (60). However, both techniques are limited
by their low energy emissions to use in superficial lesions. They
are not useful for whole body screening or evaluation of deep or
occult tumor.

67-Ga scintigraphy may be used to detect melanoma anywhere in
the body. Langhammer and associates found positive scans in 8 of
11 patients with melanoma (24). Berelowitz and co-workers had two
positive scans in four patients in their series (61).

Among 38 patients with proven melanoma studied at the NIH,
positive 67-Ga scans were obtained in 26 (14). In 10 other

patients whose tumor had been excised, nine had normal scans.
Fifty-six of 104 sites (54%) of proven involvement showed 67-Ga
accumulation. Only three of 208 sites, (2%) known to be free of
tumor, revealed 67-Ga uptake.

Melanoma masses larger than 2 cm can be visualized in 75% of
the cases, but smaller tumors are detected in only 17%. As illustrated in the accompanying examples, metastases were found in
many organs. Bone, brain, and lymph node metastases were most
reliably visualized. Both melanotic and amelanotic melanomas
could be detected. When integrated with the complete patient
work-up, the information from a 67-Ga scan can be useful in the
management of malignant melanoma. Knowledge of distant spread
of the tumor provides important prognostic information and may
obviate diagnostic surgical procedures. Negative findings on the
67-Ga scan must be considered inconclusive in the patient with
melanoma, because almost half of all lesions are missed, particularly the small ones.

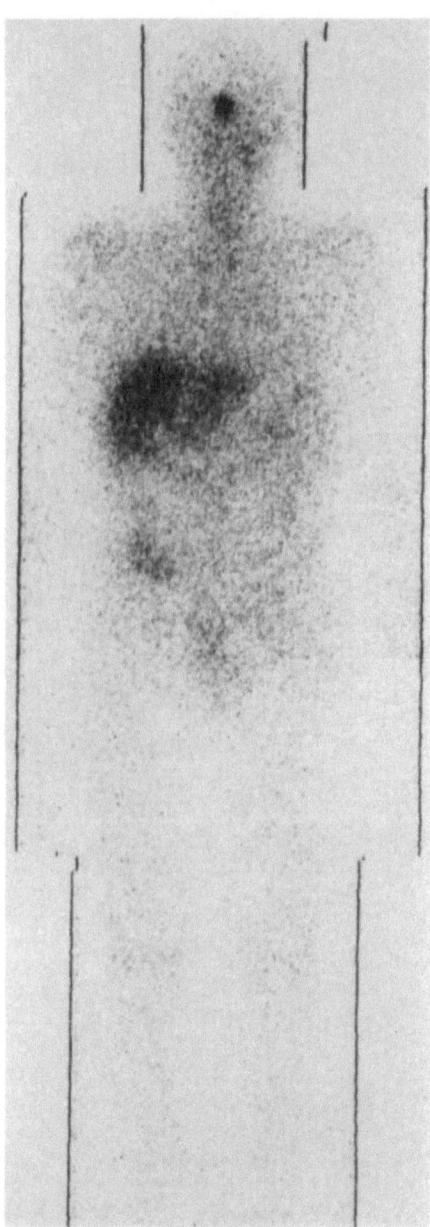

Fig. 10-1. Primary Site: A 59-year-old man was found to have slight cervical adenopathy. Excision biopsy showed metastatic malignant melanoma in a lymph node. Two months later he developed epistaxis and a primary melanoma was found on the right side of the nasal septum. The anterior 67-Ga scan obtained at that time shows intense midline facial activity at the site of the recurrent primary tumor. Recurrence was established by repeat biopsy.

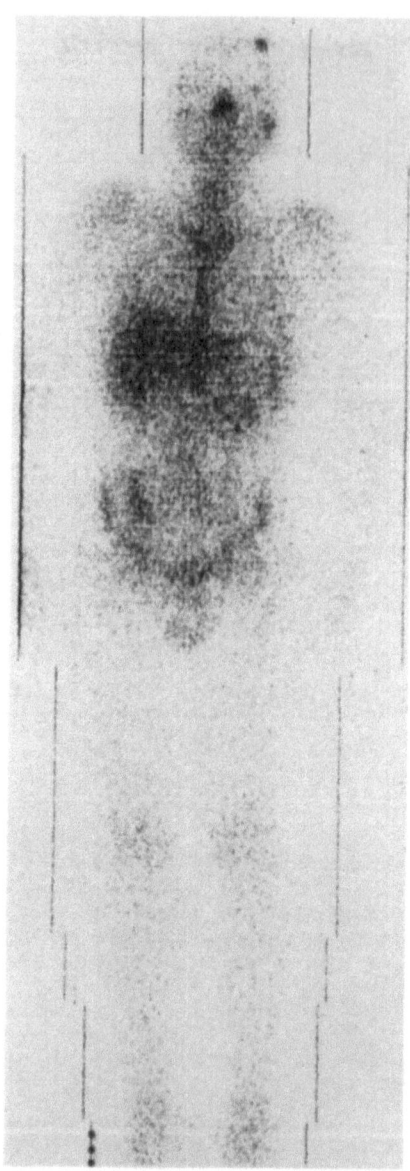

Fig. 10-2. Subcutaneous Metastases: A 29-year-old man had a
primary melanoma excised from his left leg and metastases to the
groin nodes excised soon after. Two years later he presented with
a large subcutaneous mass in the left frontal area and a palpable
left pre-auricular node. The anterior 67-Ga scan shows abnormal
activity in the left frontal area and on the left side of the face,
both superficial lesions corresponding to the clinically suspected
metastases. These were subsequently proven by biopsy to be
melanoma.

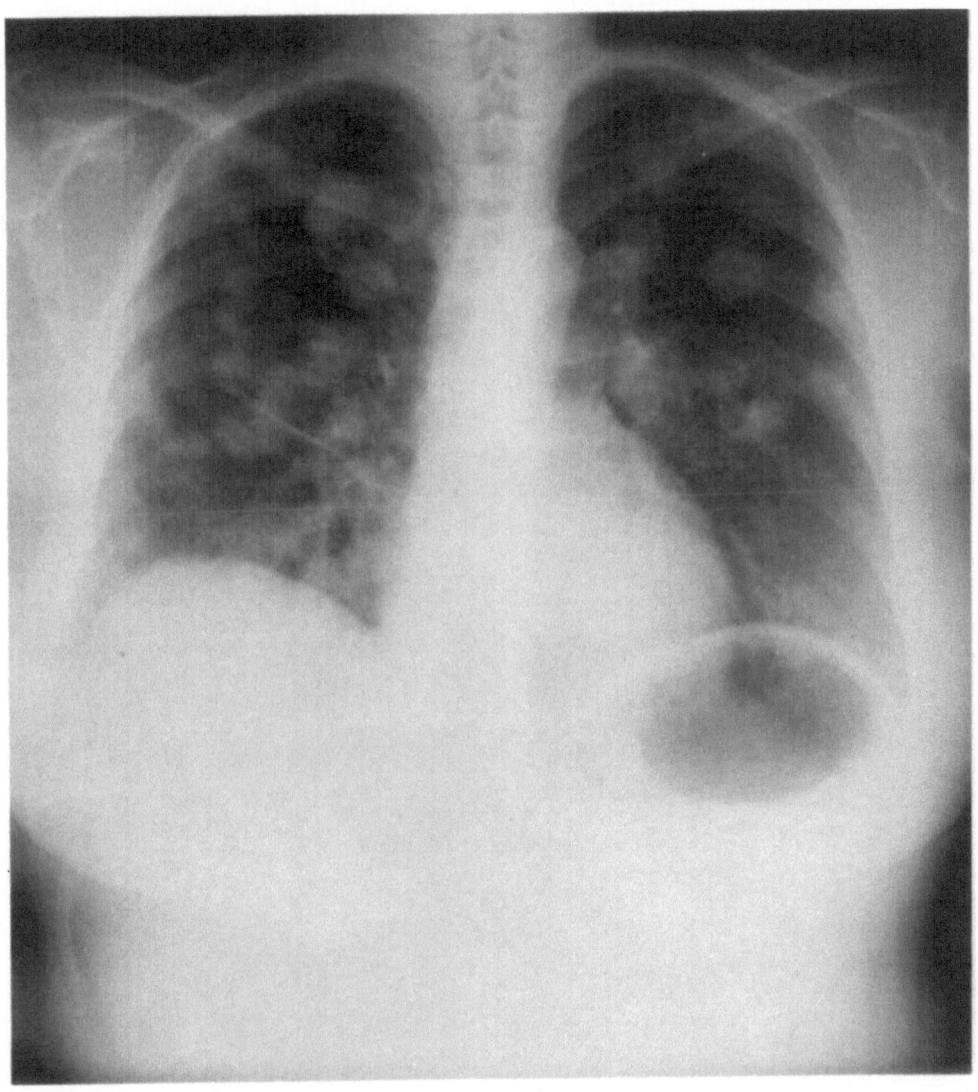

Fig. 10-3A. Lung and Brain Metastases: A 43-year-old woman had a two-year history of melanoma with pulmonary metastases resistant to multiple chemotherapeutic regimens. Two weeks before admission she developed headache. The PA chest roentgenogram shows numerous round masses throughout both lungs.

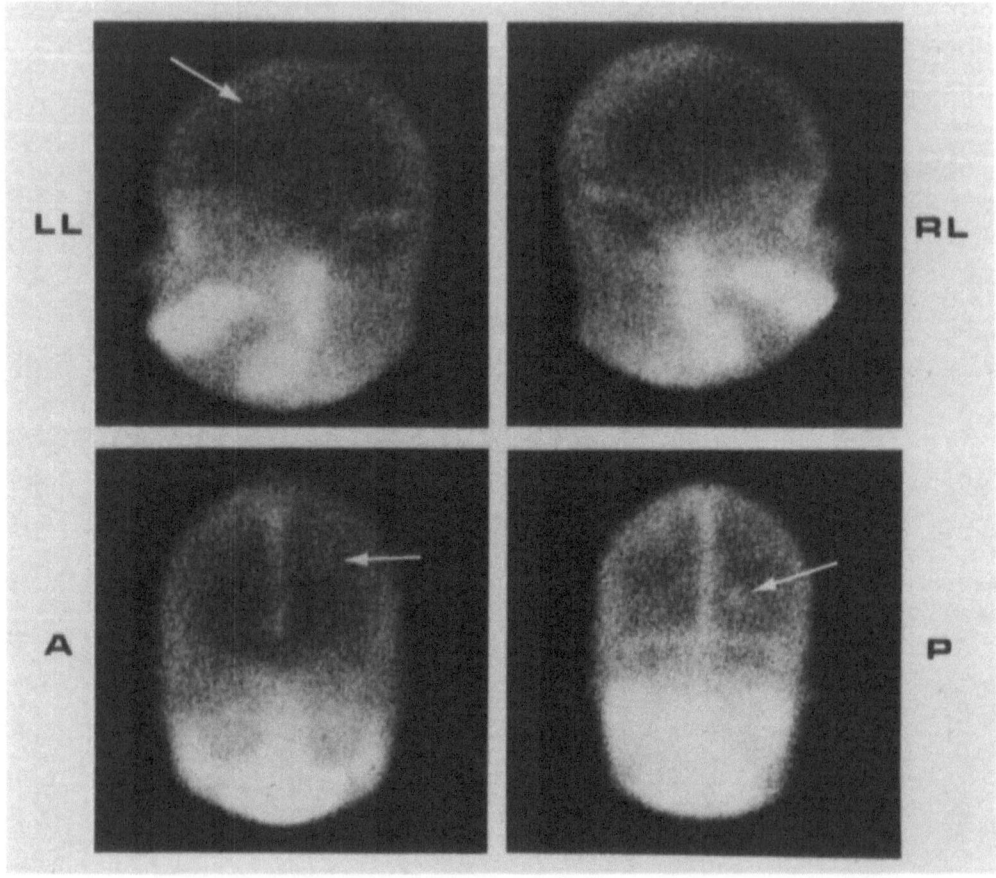

Fig. 10-3B. Lung and Brain Metastases (continued): A 99m-Tc
pertechnetate brain scan shows abnormal activity in the left
frontal region and the right occipital area (arrows). LL = left
lateral; RL = right lateral; A = anterior; P = posterior.

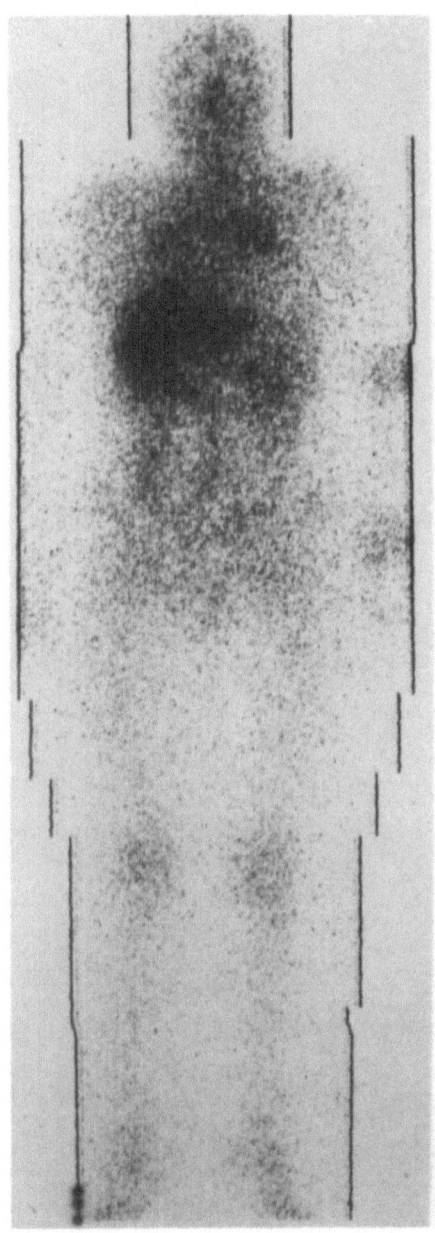 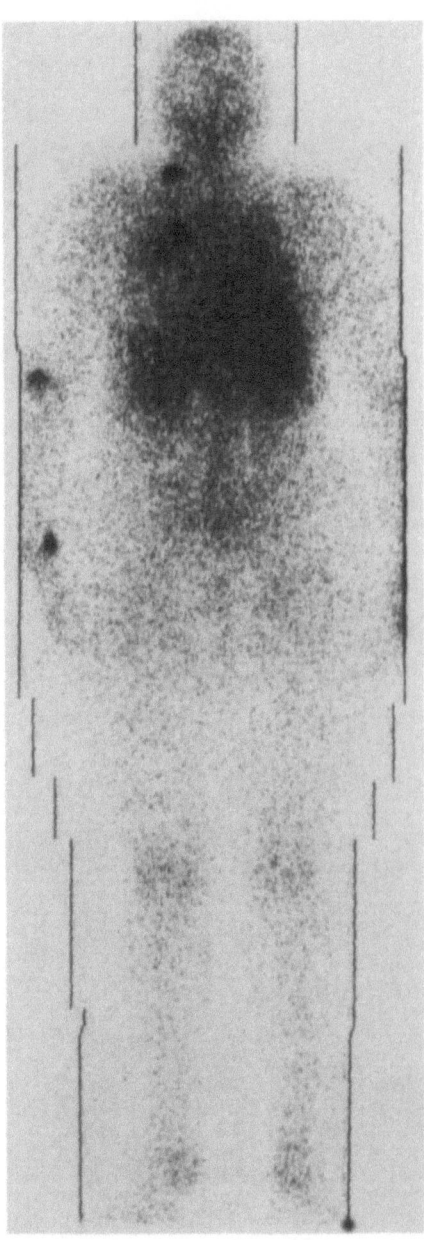

Fig. 10-3C. Lung and Brain Metastases (continued): 67-Ga scans
demonstrated intense uptake in both lungs and in a posterior cervical
node as well as faint activity in the brain lesions. Foci in the
left arm are injection sites. The patient rapidly developed
increased intracranial pressure and died of cerebral herniation.
At autopsy multiple 1-3 cm pulmonary metastases and bilateral
cerebral melanomas were found.

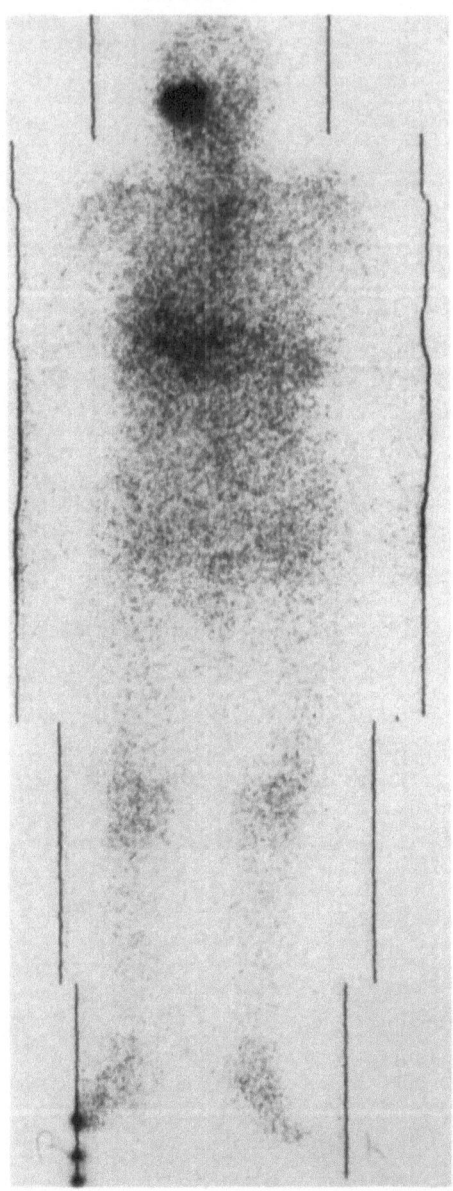

Fig. 10-4. Bone Involvement: An 80-year-old woman developed
fullness in the right cheek and an elevated right eye. Examination
revealed a mass in the right nasal cavity. Radiologic studies
showed a large mass in the right maxillary antrum with destruction
of the maxillary and ethmoid sinuses on the right. Aspiration of
the maxillary sinus yielded melanoma cells. The anterior 67-Ga
scan shows an intense accumulation on the right side of the face
corresponding to the proven destructive tumor.

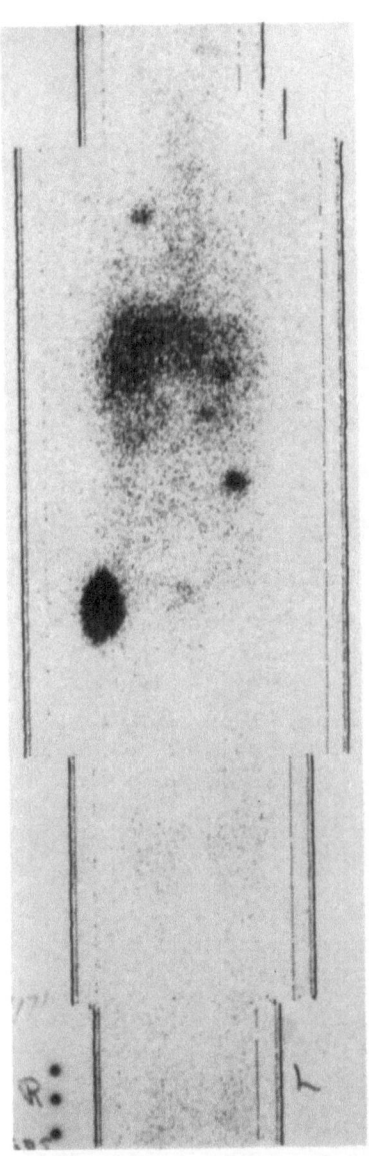 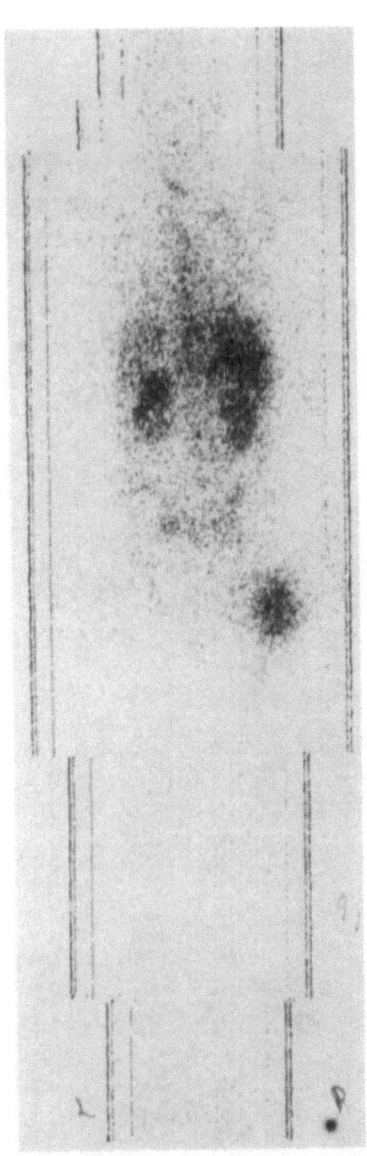

Fig. 10-5. Metastases to Kidney: A 25-year-old man with xeroderma pigmentosa had a four-year history of malignant melanoma with wide-spread metastases to the skin, nodes and viscera. He developed dark urine and urine cytology revealed melanoma cells. The posterior 67-Ga scan shows uniform uptake in both kidneys. In addition, there is a large right hip lesion. The anterior view shows the hip lesion, multiple abdominal and chest foci, and a left cerebral tumor. The patient died two months later of massive pulmonary emboli. Autopsy confirmed bilateral renal melanoma as well as large metastases to the brain, lung, bowel, hip, and testes, and many small metastases.

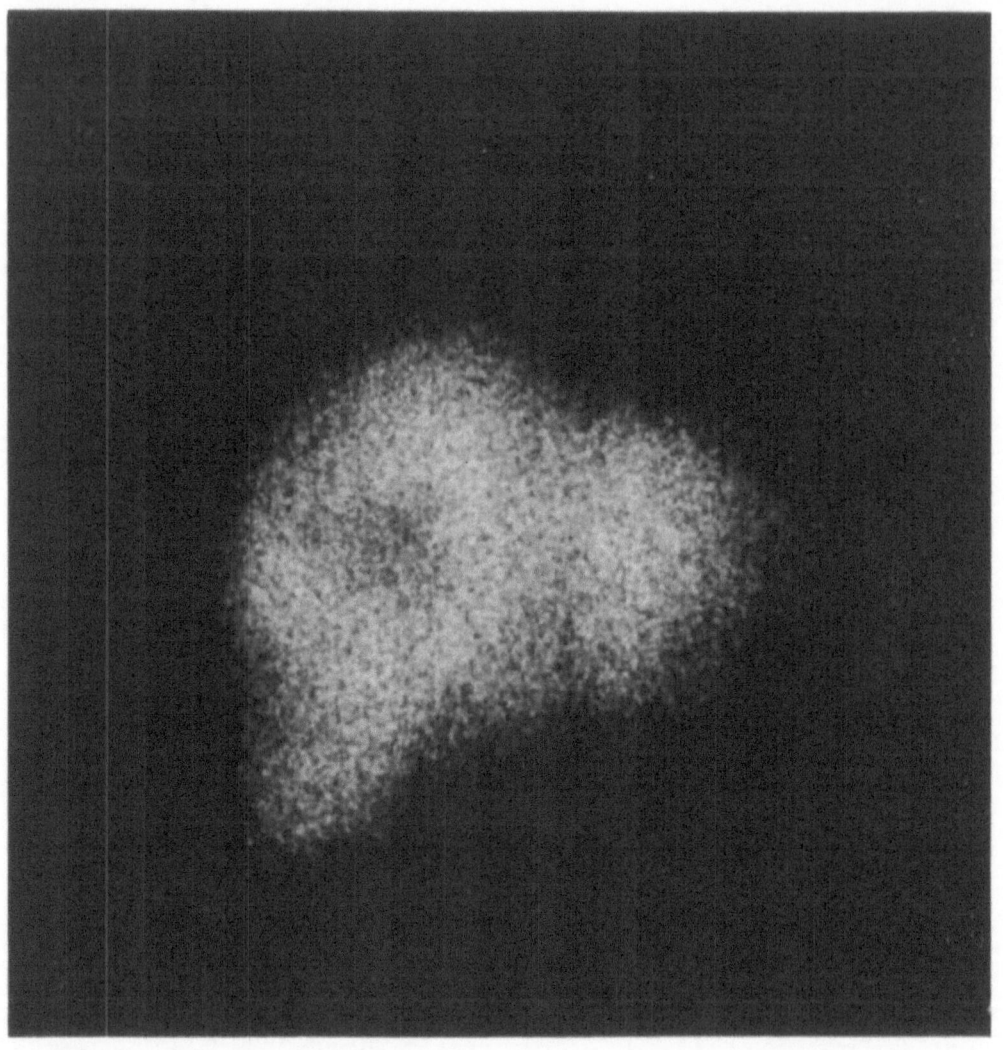

Fig. 10-6A. Liver Metastases: A 16-year-old girl had an apparently benign mole excised two years before admission and later developed numerous subcutaneous nodules which were melanoma on biopsy. A chest x-ray showed pulmonary metastases. A 99m-Tc sulfur colloid liver scan shows an area of decreased uptake of isotope in the mid-right lobe.

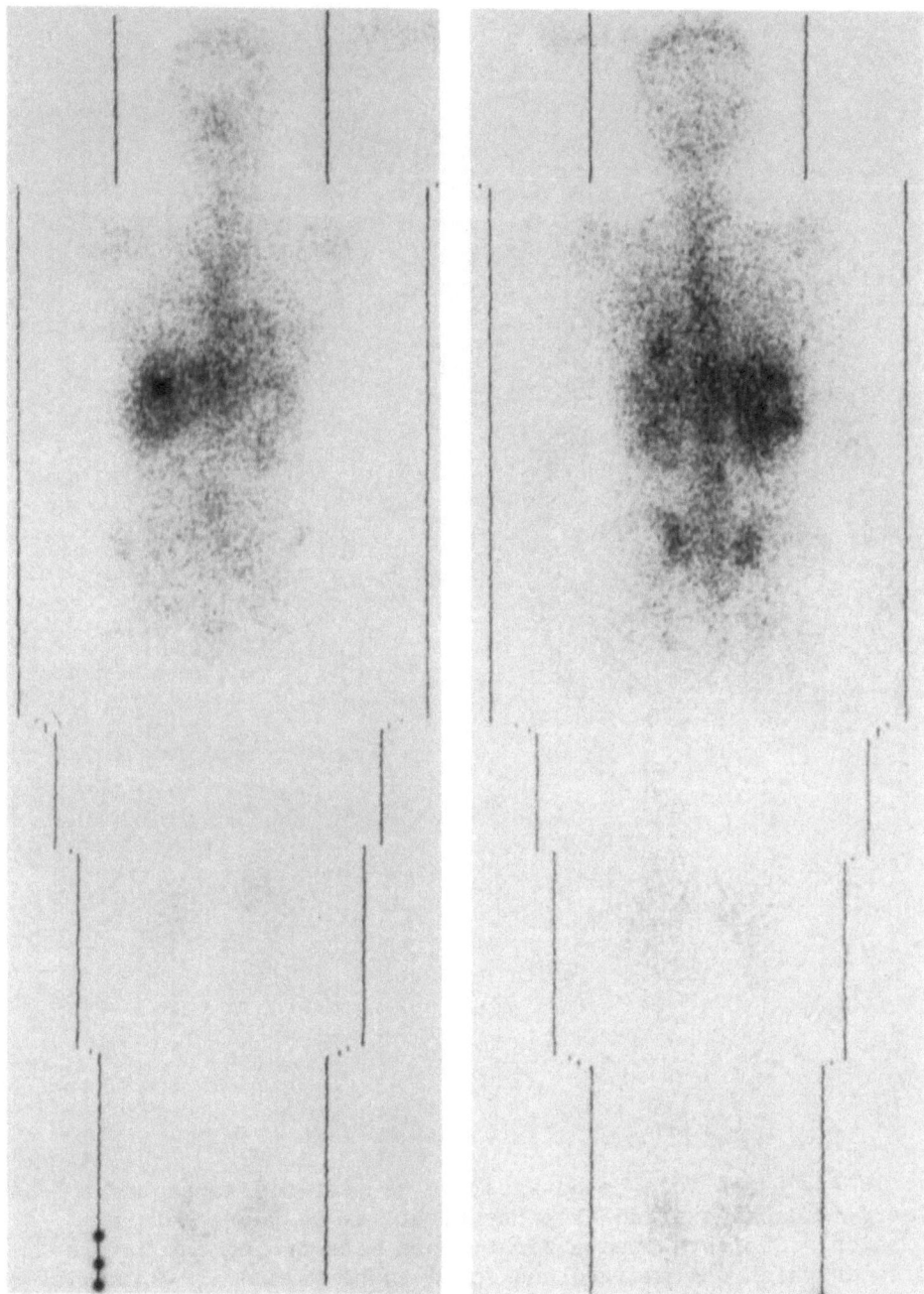

Fig. 10-6B.   Liver Metastases (continued): The 67-Ga scan shows
a corresponding area of uptake in the liver. The posterior view
shows two lesions in the liver and a discrete mass at the left
lung base.

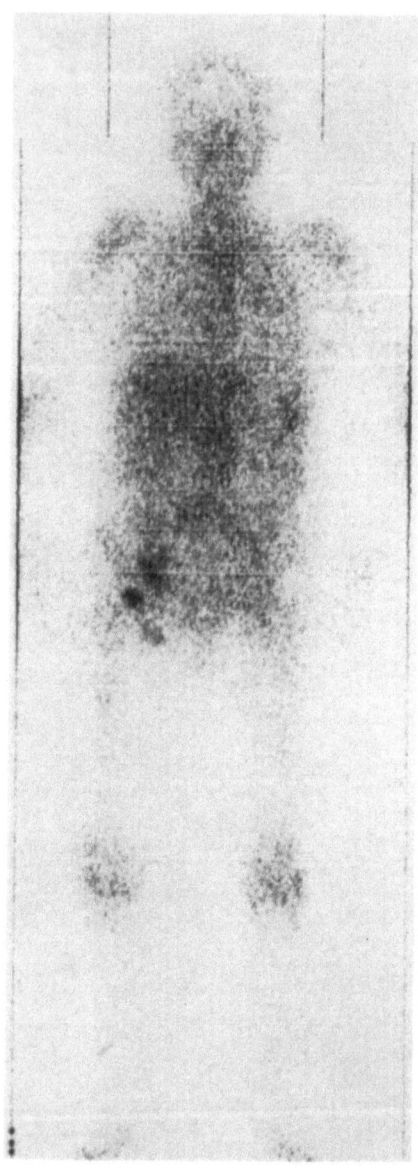

Fig. 10-7. Lymph Node Metastases: A 61-year-old woman had a
primary melanoma excised from her right leg 14 years before
admission. She developed a right groin mass two months before
admission which was excised and found to be melanoma. On admission
she had 3 cm masses in the right iliac, inguinal and femoral
regions. A 67-Ga scan shows three discrete foci of uptake in the
right groin corresponding to the three palpable masses. No evidence
of the primary tumor remains. A left scalene node biopsy revealed
metastatic melanoma and no further surgery was done.

CHAPTER 11

Brain Tumors

Alfred E. Jones, M. D.

Department of Nuclear Medicine, Clinical Center

National Institutes of Health, Bethesda, Maryland

In 1971, physicians at NIH proposed that the recognized
specificity of 67-Ga, for many forms of neoplasia, might be used in
conjunction with 99m-Tc pertechnetate for the detection of intracranial tumors (62,67). It was necessary to define a method for
performing 67-Ga brain studies and then to compare its usefulness,
in the detection of intracranial tumors, with the established brain
scintigraphic technique utilizing 99m-Tc pertechnetate. This
comparative approach was initiated by selecting patients who were
known to have primary brain tumors and positive 99m-Tc brain studies
and then comparing the 67-Ga images of the same lesion. Later,
99m-Tc polyphosphate was used to evaluate skull lesions (surgical
and metastatic) along with 67-Ga images and 99m-Tc pertechnetate
images.

In the method adopted, images were collected on polaroid film
30 to 60 minutes after the intravenous administration of 15 mCi of
99m-Tc pertechnetate. Three hundred thousand counts were obtained
for each view and on completion of this aspect of the study, 67-Ga
was administered intravenously, 50 µCi/kg body weight. Images were
collected on polaroid film, 48 to 72 hours later, gathering fifty
thousand counts per view and utilizing a high energy collimator in
contrast to the low energy, high resolution collimator used with the
99m-Tc pertechnetate study. The gamma camera energy range was set
at 190 Kev. Although brain images may be collected before 24 hours
have elapsed (Fig. 11-2), an optimal qualitative localization appears
to take place by 48 to 72 hours.

The 67-Ga brain scintigraph is similar to the 99m-Tc pertechnetate image insofar as there is normally more activity seen in the

161

areas representing the skull and face than in the area of the
brain. A bilaterally symmetrical increase in 67-Ga activity may
be seen in the region of the lacrimal glands and thus far has not
been related to any pathologic state. Unlike 99m-Tc, 67-Ga shows
no increased localization of activity in the mouth and usually a
minimal increase in the salivary glands. In addition, 67-Ga does
not accumulate in the choroid plexus. Individuals may have an
increase in 67-Ga in the region of the nasopharynx while the nose
itself rarely shows more activity than the surrounding facial
structures (Fig. 11-1).

Primary brain tumors were studied preoperatively and postoperatively. In both situations certain of the 67-Ga studies were
abnormal when the 99m-Tc pertechnetate views were interpreted as
being normal. In the postoperative period, 67-Ga brain scintigraphy
has been helpful in resolving tumor from the previous craniotomy
site (Fig. 11-3 and 11-4). The addition of 99m-Tc polyphosphate
skull scintigraphy has further refined the delineation of the
craniotomy site from recurrent tumor. When the 99m-Tc pertechnetate
brain images are abnormal in the months and years after craniotomy,
the 67-Ga images may distinguish the area of existing neoplasm
from the diffusely localized activity of 99m-Tc pertechnetate in the
bone flap induced by the preceding craniotomy (Fig. 11-4).

67-Ga brain scintigraphy has produced negative results after
primary brain tumors or metastatic brain lesions have been treated
by radiation (Fig. 7-13C) and/or chemotherapy. Following treatment,
99m-Tc pertechnetate brain scintigraphy may result in a positive
study while 67-Ga may reveal little or no abnormality (Fig. 11-5).
It is uncertain whether or not this is due to suppression of the
neoplasm or inability of the tumor to take up 67-Ga due to a change
induced by the preceding therapy or a combination of the two (Fig.
11-5). The value of 67-Ga brain scintigraphy remains uncertain in
this situation.

Brain scintigraphy with 67-Ga has been especially helpful in
delineating metastatic brain lesions (63). Frequently, these
metastases are more clearly delineated by 67-Ga than by 99m-Tc
pertechnetate (Figs. 11-8 and 11-12) and occasionally lesions are
detected with 67-Ga that have not been observed on the 99m-Tc
pertechnetate brain study (Fig. 11-9). This latter situation has
also been observed when there are metastases to the skull and
99m-Tc pertechnetate studies have been interpreted as normal. In
this instance, the 99m-Tc polyphosphate views of the head (skull)
will reveal the skull lesions as well but will not detect the
intracranial lesions that are clearly shown by 67-Ga. Occasionally,
99m-Tc polyphosphate will be observed to localize faintly in an
intracranial lesion. In each of these instances, the 99m-Tc
pertechnetate study has been clearly abnormal and the 67-Ga
localization has been strongly positive (Fig. 11-10).

67-Ga has localized in benign lesions of the scalp and skull (Figs. 11-13 and 11-14). The quantity of the 67-Ga localized in these abnormalities has been significantly less than in neoplastic lesions where there is frequently an intense accumulation of 67-Ga.

67-Ga brain scintigraphy has proven useful in the detection of brain tumors; assessment of brain tumor recurrence; and evaluation of suspected metastatic brain lesions. The 67-Ga procedure is not intended to replace 99m-Tc pertechnetate brain scintigraphy but should serve as a useful supplement. The procedure may be conveniently accomplished following the 67-Ga whole body rectilinear survey for metastatic lesions.

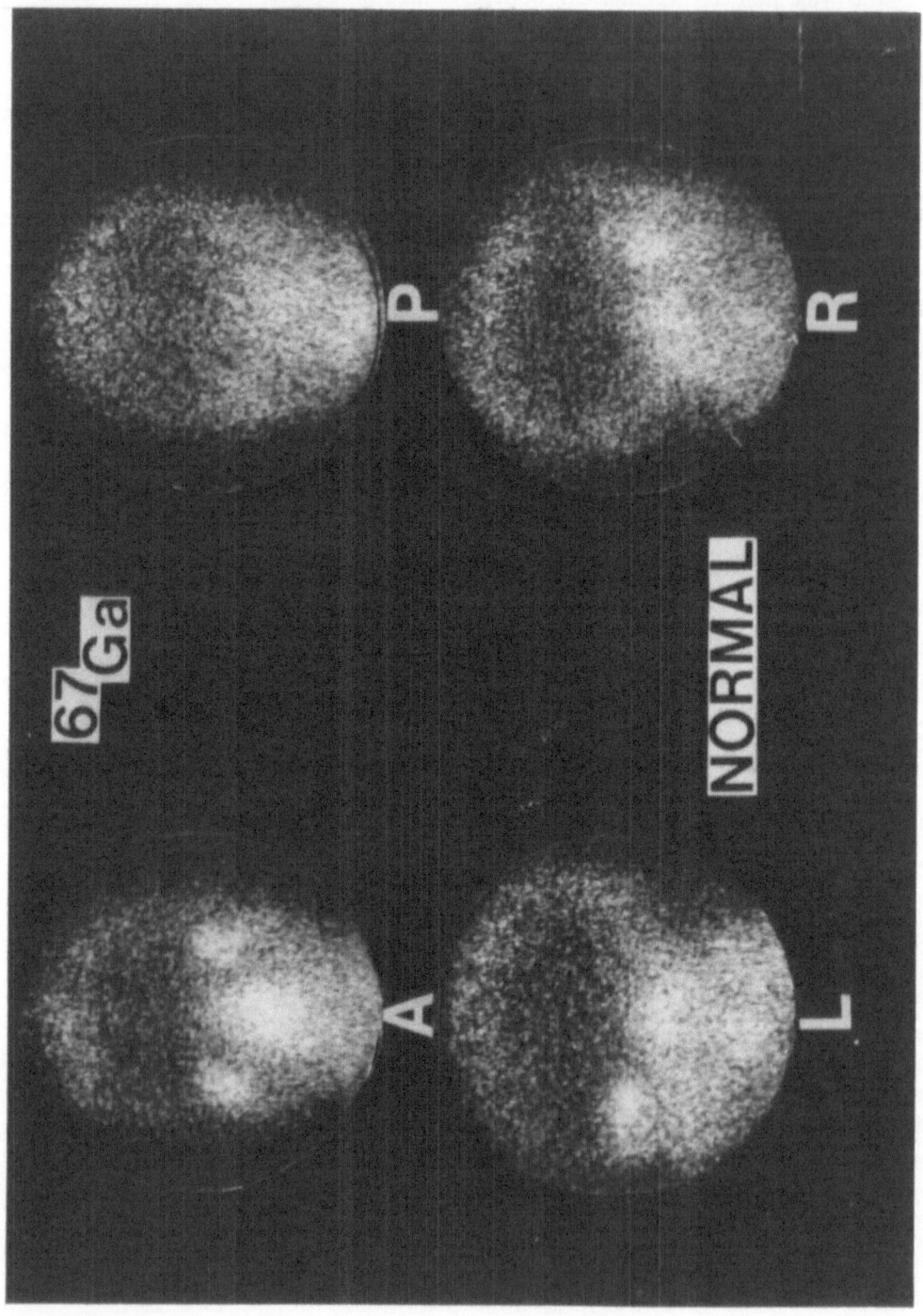

Fig. 11-1. Normal 67-Ga scintigraphs at 48 to 72 hours represent the brain as a region of low activity in comparison to the skull and facial areas. Major differences between the 67-Ga and the 99m-Tc pertechnetate brain scintigraphs are: absence of 67-Ga concentration in the choroid plexus and salivary glands; non-visualization of the lateral vascular sinuses; a variable increase in 67-Ga activity in the lacrimal glands of both normal and abnormal subjects; a faintly visible sagittal sinus and a prominent localization of 67-Ga in the nasopharynx. Note that on the lateral views the lacrimal glands appear to be in the low temporal area. L = left; A = anterior; P = posterior; R = right.

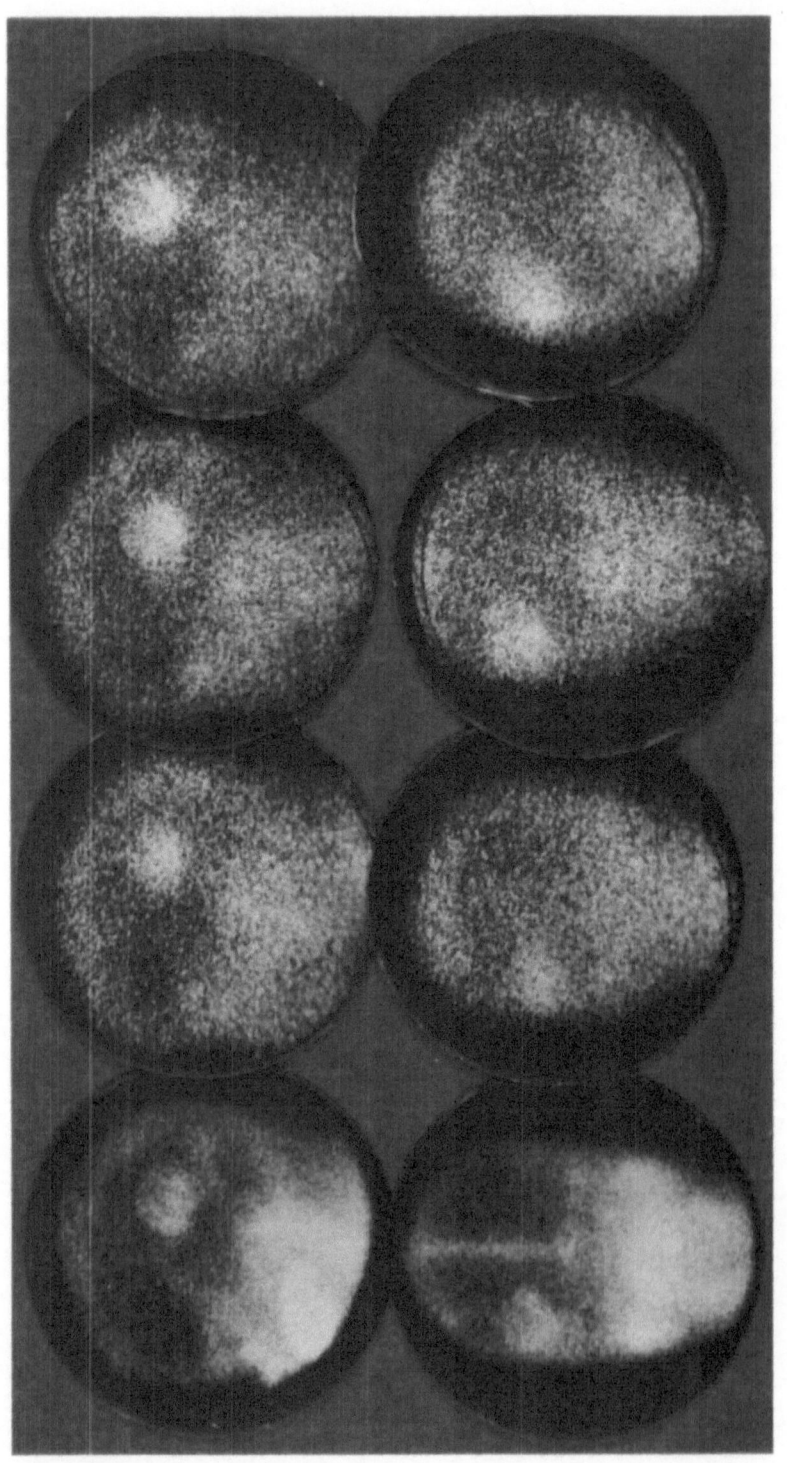

Fig. 11-2. 99m-Tc pertechnetate and 67-Ga brain studies of 14-year-old girl with a grade IV cystic glioblastoma of the left mid-temporal lobe. The patient had a craniotomy and radiation therapy one year prior to scan. Top row, left lateral views; bottom row, posterior views. Both rows from left to right: 99m-Tc pertechnetate; 67-Ga 16-hour views; 24-hour views; and 48-hour views. Note that the size of the lesion in 99m-Tc pertechnetate images is similar to the size on subsequent 67-Ga images.

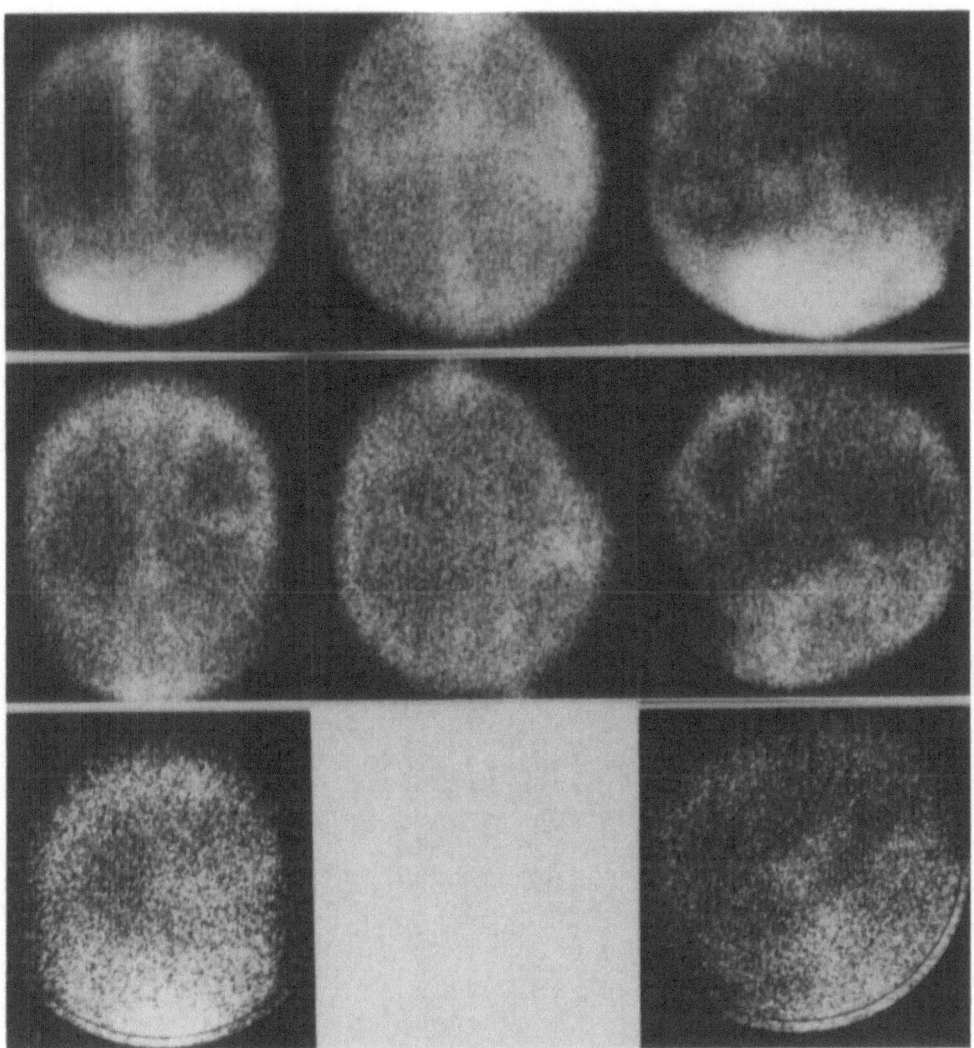

Fig. 11-3. Post Craniotomy Study: Sixty-year-old woman with a
large right parietal glioblastoma multiforme and left hemiparesis.
Craniotomy performed 29 days before 99m-Tc pertechnetate study; 32
days before 67-Ga views; and 43 days prior to 99m-Tc polyphosphate
scintigraphy. Left to right: posterior, vertex, right lateral.
Note craniotomy site outlined in 99m-Tc polyphosphate views (middle
row, across). Tumor is seen in the posterior and right lateral
67-Ga views (lower row) while both tumor and operative site are
seen in the 99m-Tc pertechnetate images (top row). In cases where
the cranial operative site and neoplasm have been superimposed in
the 99m-Tc pertechnetate views, it has been helpful to obtain 67-Ga
brain scintigraphs. The above study was chosen for demonstration
because of the separate locations of neoplasm and operative site.

P   R

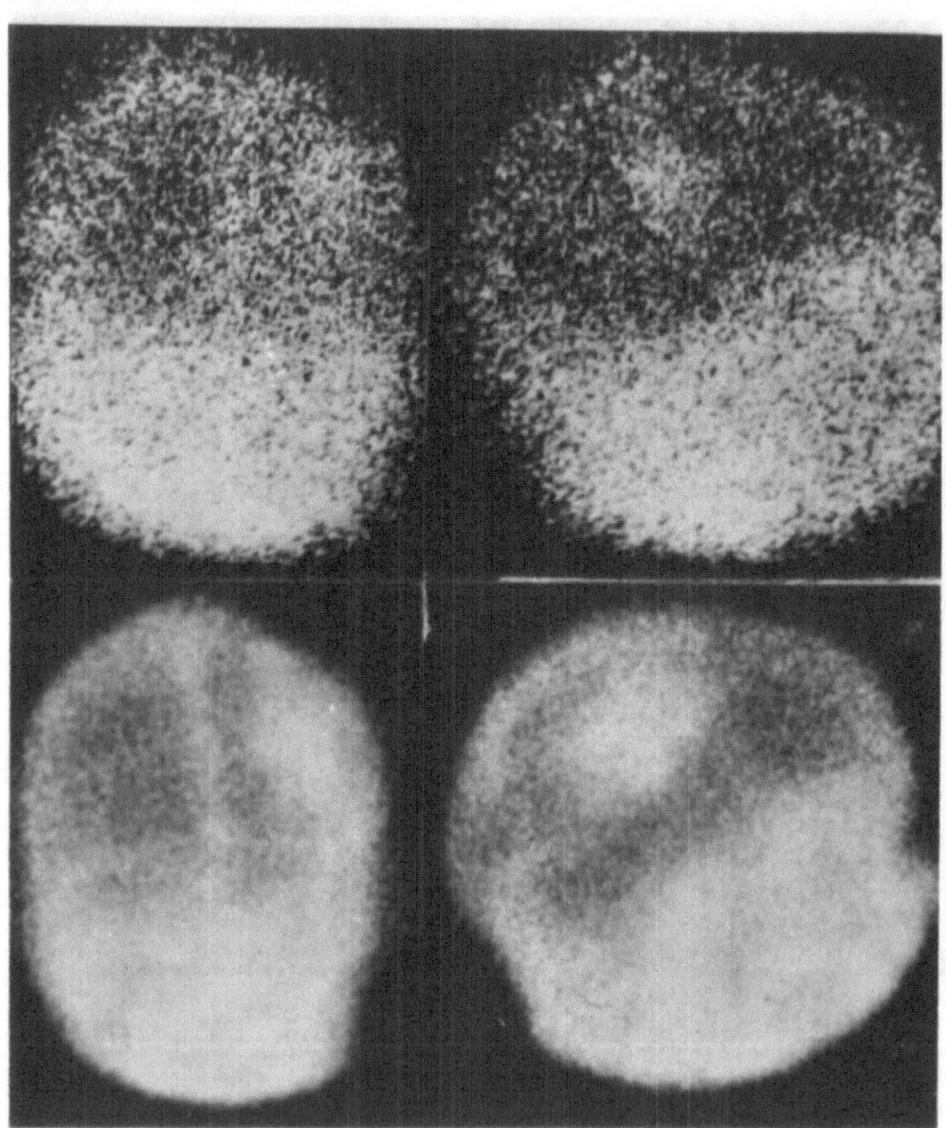

Fig. 11-4. 67-Ga (above) and 99m-Tc pertechnetate (below);
posterior and right lateral views of a 41-year-old woman with a
two-year history of a right parietal lobe grade III astrocytoma.
The patient had a craniotomy 12 months previously and subsequent
chemotherapy. Note that the area of abnormality is larger on the
99m-Tc pertechnetate study than on the 67-Ga study. The former
study delineated operative site and remaining neoplasm while 67-Ga
defined the remaining tumor. P = posterior, R = right.

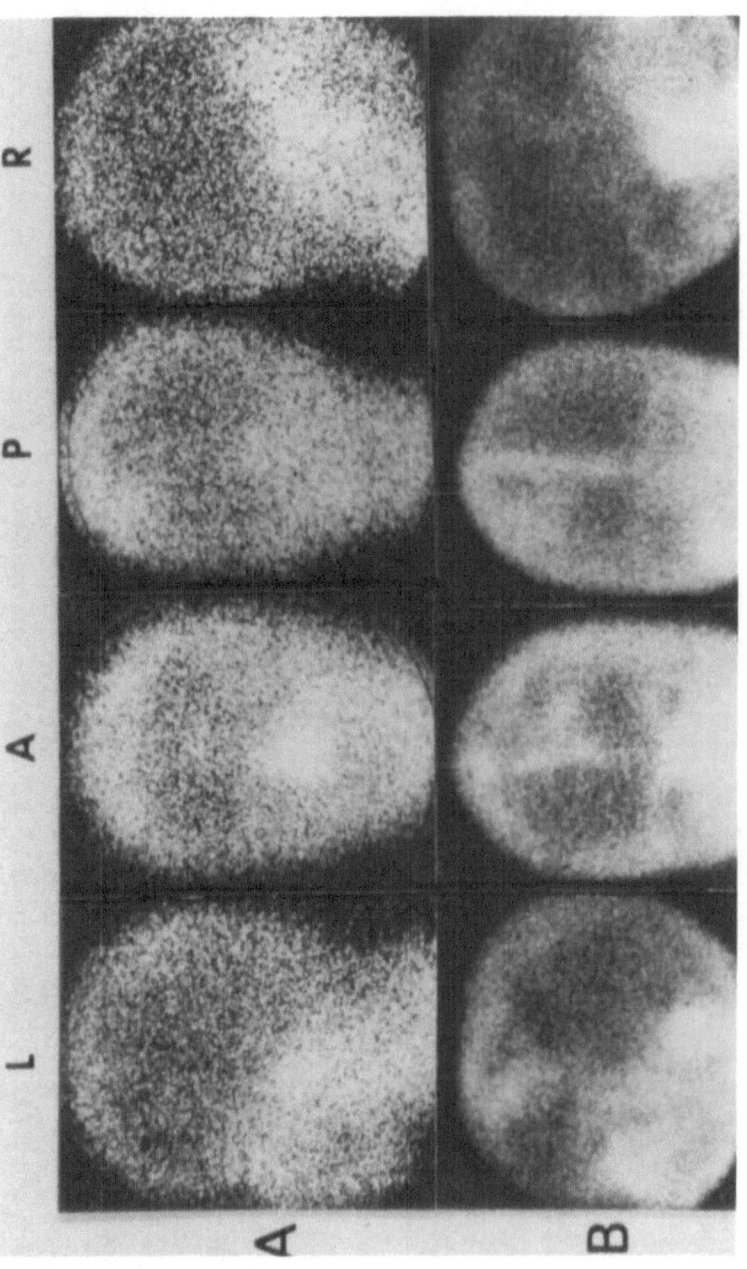

Fig. 11-5. 67-Ga (top) and 99m-Tc pertechnetate studies (bottom) of a 28-year-old woman with a grade III astrocytoma. The patient underwent craniotomy, radiation therapy and chemotherapy prior to scintigraphy. An Ommaya reservoir is in place through which chemotherapy was administered. There is poor localization of 67-Ga in the area of the tumor. Lack of 67-Ga localization within tumor is frequently observed after radiation or chemotherapy. The abnormality seen on the 99m-Tc pertechnetate study relates to the previous craniotomy and implantation of the reservoir. L = left; A = anterior; P = posterior; R = right.

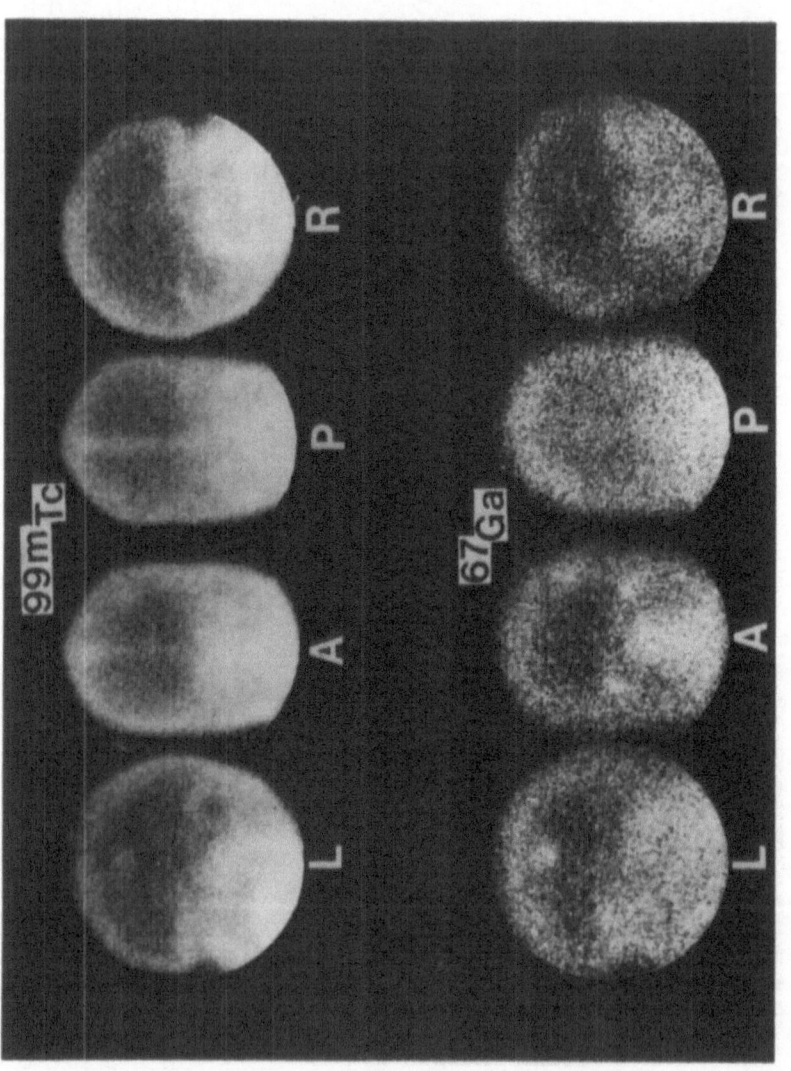

Fig. 11-6. Metastatic epidermoid carcinoma in the left parietal area not seen on a 99m-Tc pertechnetate study obtained 5 weeks previously. The above 67-Ga views were obtained within 3 days of the 99m-Tc pertechnetate views shown. Scintigraphy was performed before the lesion was treated. The lesion is seen more distinctly with 67-Ga and appears equal in size with 99m-Tc pertechnetate. Both lacrimal glands are clearly seen in the appropriate 67-Ga views. L = left; A = anterior; P = posterior; R = right.

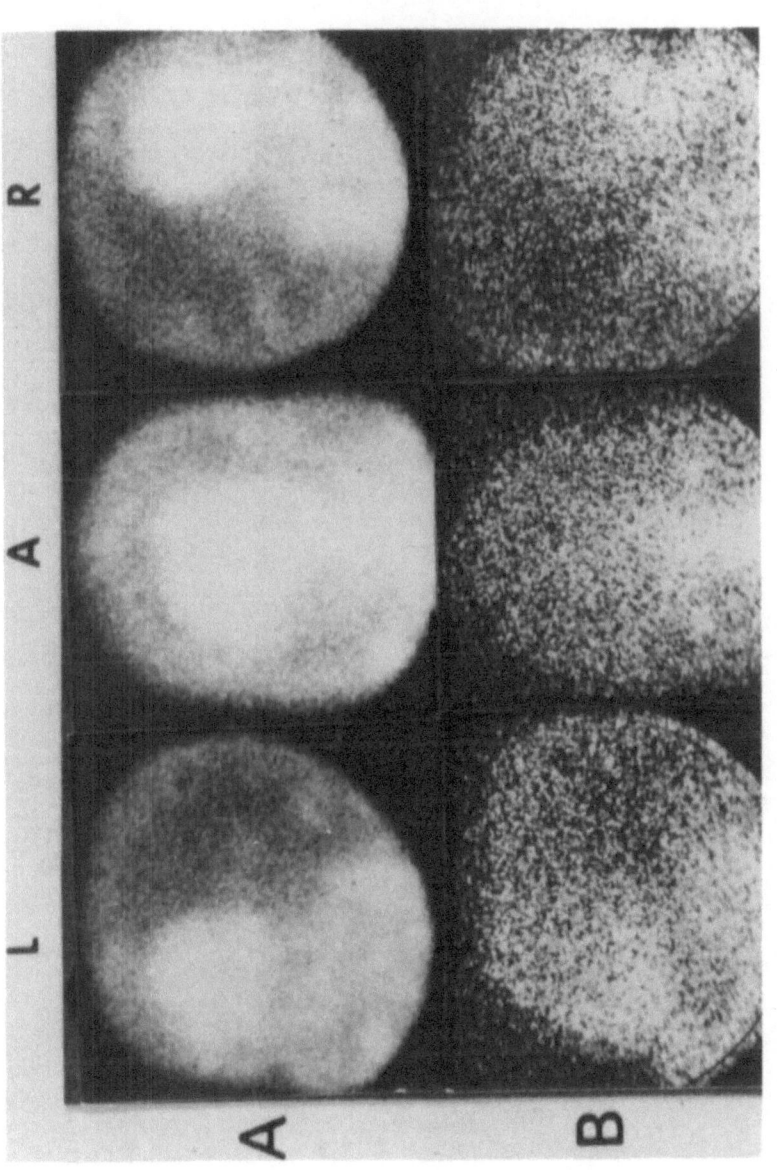

Fig. 11-7. Metastatic bronchial adenoma involving left and right anterior cerebral hemispheres of a 33-year-old man. Craniotomy and surgical resection of the tumor was performed on three occasions. He also had radiation therapy and chemotherapy. 99m-Tc pertechnetate (top row) clearly demonstrates the magnitude of the tumor while the 67-Ga (bottom row) views indicate poor tumor localization. The 99m-Tc pertechnetate defines both the tumor and the operative site. The lack of significant 67-Ga localization may be due to prior radiation and chemotherapy of this metastatic brain tumor. L = left; A = anterior; R = right.

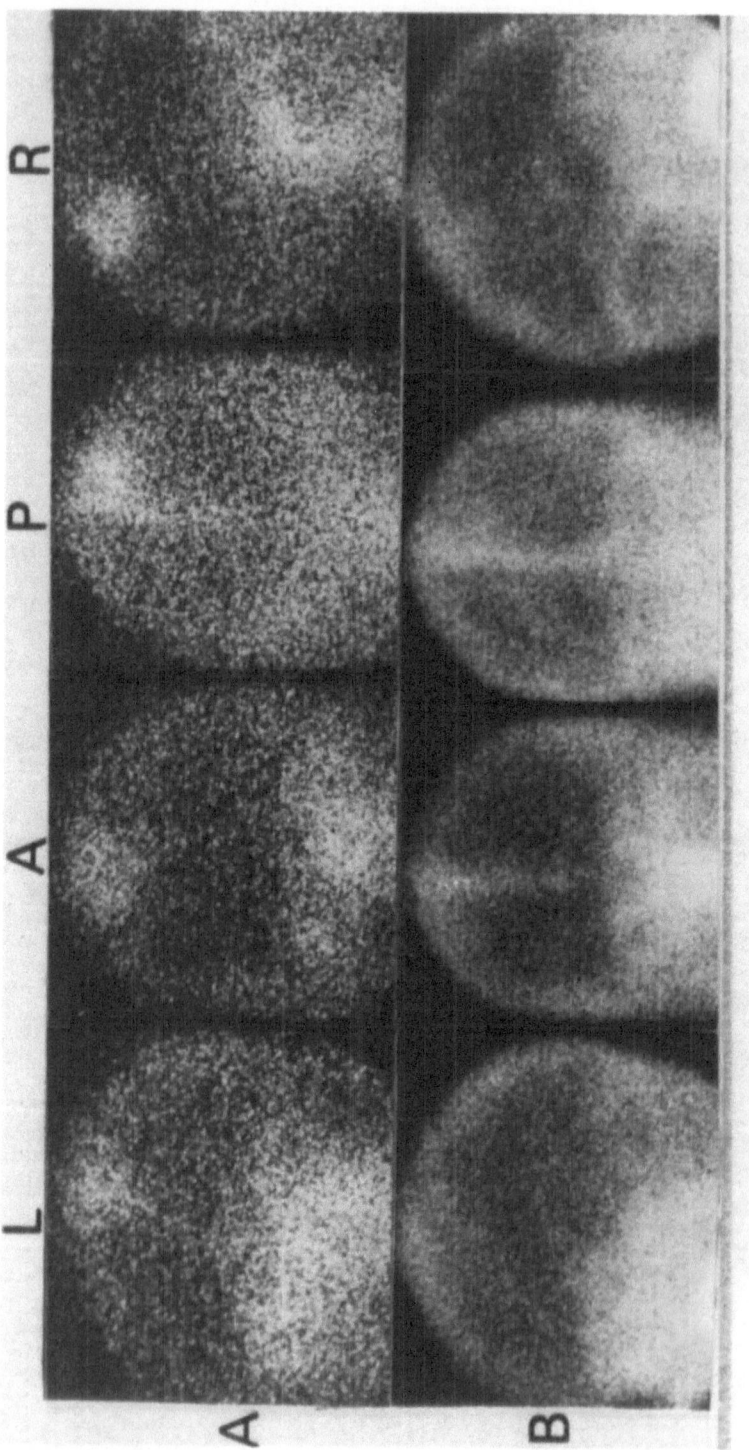

Fig. 11-8. Malignant lymphoma metastatic to the right posterior parietal area in a 54-year-old man with clinical findings of cerebral involvement (see Fig. 7-12B). 67-Ga (top row) clearly defined the metastasis which is much less clearly seen with 99m-Tc pertechnetate (bottom row). L = left; A = anterior; P = posterior; R = right.

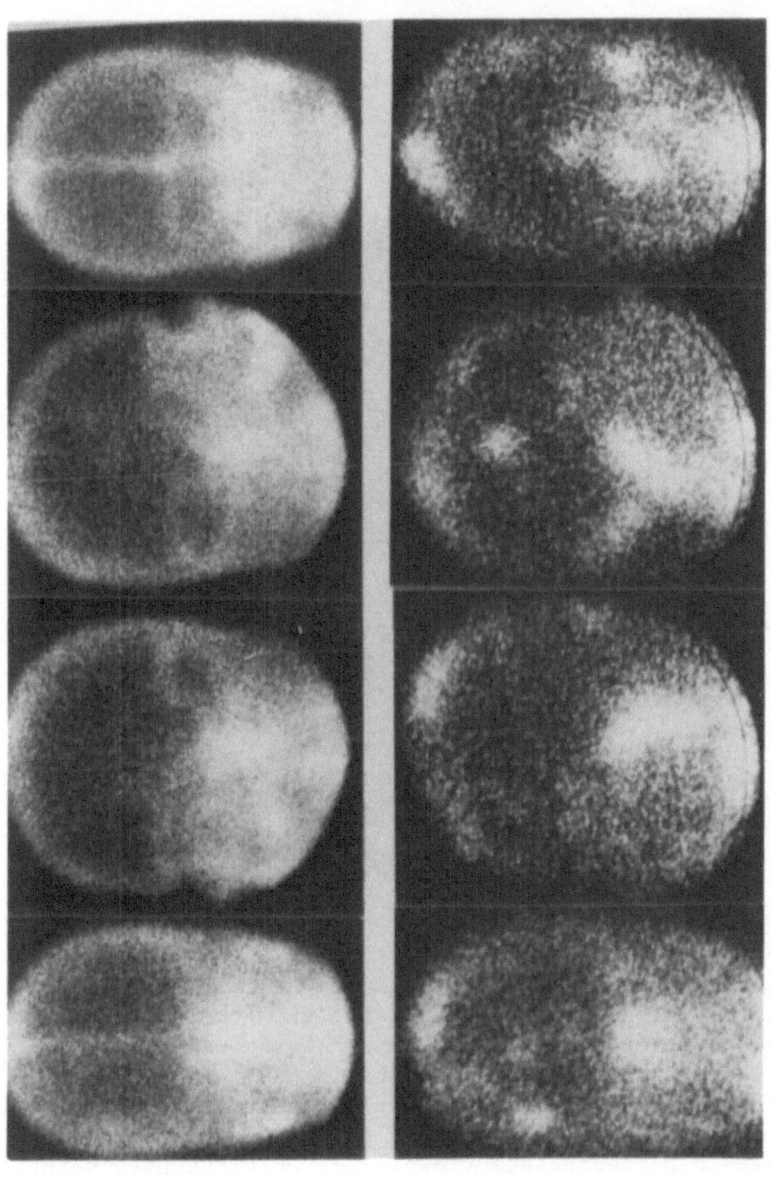

Fig. 11-9. 99m-Tc pertechnetate (top row) and 67-Ga (bottom row) brain scintigraphs of a 34-year-old man with Hodgkin's disease. History and whole body scans are described in Fig. 7-5. The 99m-Tc pertechnetate scintigraphs appear strikingly benign in comparison to the 67-Ga scintigraphs which show multiple cranial lesions. The whole body scans of the patient (Fig. 7-5B and C) show the cranial involvement but the extent is not evident by the rectilinear technique. It is helpful to obtain gamma camera views of the head immediately following the rectilinear study.

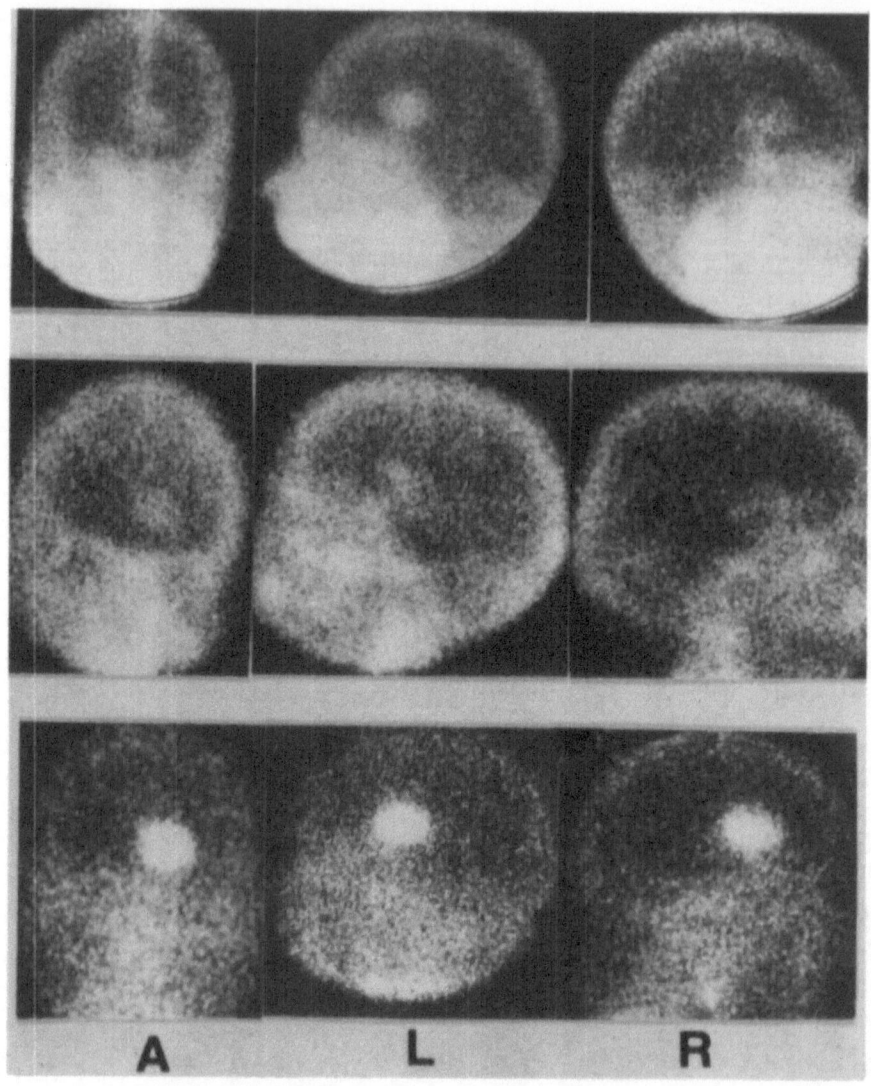

Fig. 11-10. Malignant lymphoma metastatic to the left cerebral
hemisphere of a 65-year-old man. The patient was studied with
99m-Tc pertechnetate (top), 99m-Tc polyphosphate (middle), and
67-Ga (lower). Note that: (1) The metastasis has not involved
the cranium and demonstrates an exceptional affinity for 67-Ga.
(2) The lesion is less distinctly seen in the 99m-Tc polyphosphate
views and the 99m-Tc pertechnetate views. (3) Polyphosphate scintigraphs have rarely showed metastasis to the cerebrum. (4) The
latter were obtained in conjunction with a whole body rectilinear
scintigraphic survey for bone lesions (Figs. 7-13A; 7-13B). (5)
Serial 67-Ga gamma camera scintigrams were obtained during radiation
therapy (Fig. 7-13C). A = anterior; L = left; R = right.

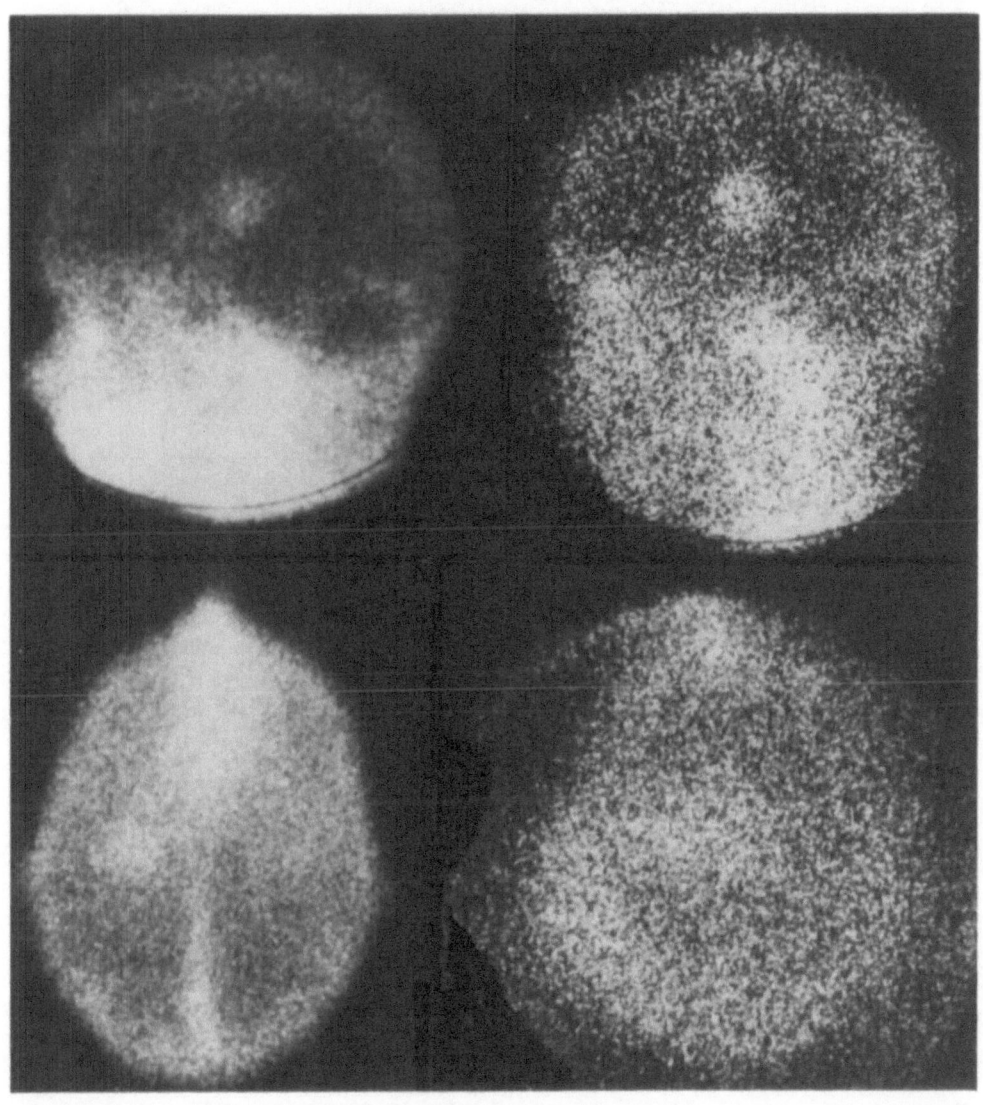

Fig. 11-11. Left lateral and vertex brain scintigraphs performed
with 99m-Tc pertechnetate (left) and 67-Ga (right) on a 44-year-old
woman with metastatic cancer of the breast and a progressive right
hemiparesis. A deep metastatic lesion is well demonstrated by both
nuclides and appears equal in size when studied by either technique.
This is in contrast to Fig. 11-9 where metastatic lesions in the
cranial vault are seen only with 67-Ga.

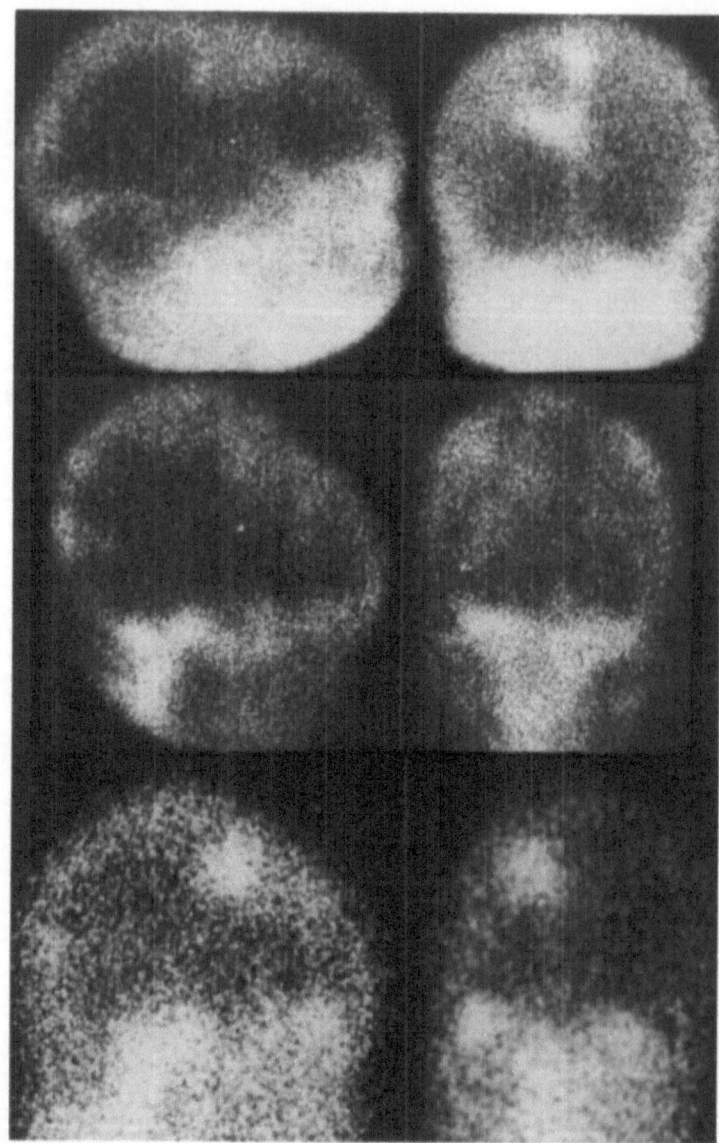

Fig. 11-12. Metastatic breast carcinoma to the cranium and cerebrum
is demonstrated on right lateral and anterior gamma camera scintigraphs utilizing 99m-Tc pertechnetate (top), 99m-Tc polyphosphate
(middle), and 67-Ga (bottom). Note the different appearance of the
lesion with each radiopharmaceutical used. The intense localization
of 67-Ga clearly defines the metastatic lesion. The 99m-Tc polyphosphate, in addition to revealing the cranial involvement at the
site of the tumor, also detects a wider range of alteration in the
bone of the cranial vault than observed on either the 67-Ga or
99m-Tc pertechnetate studies.

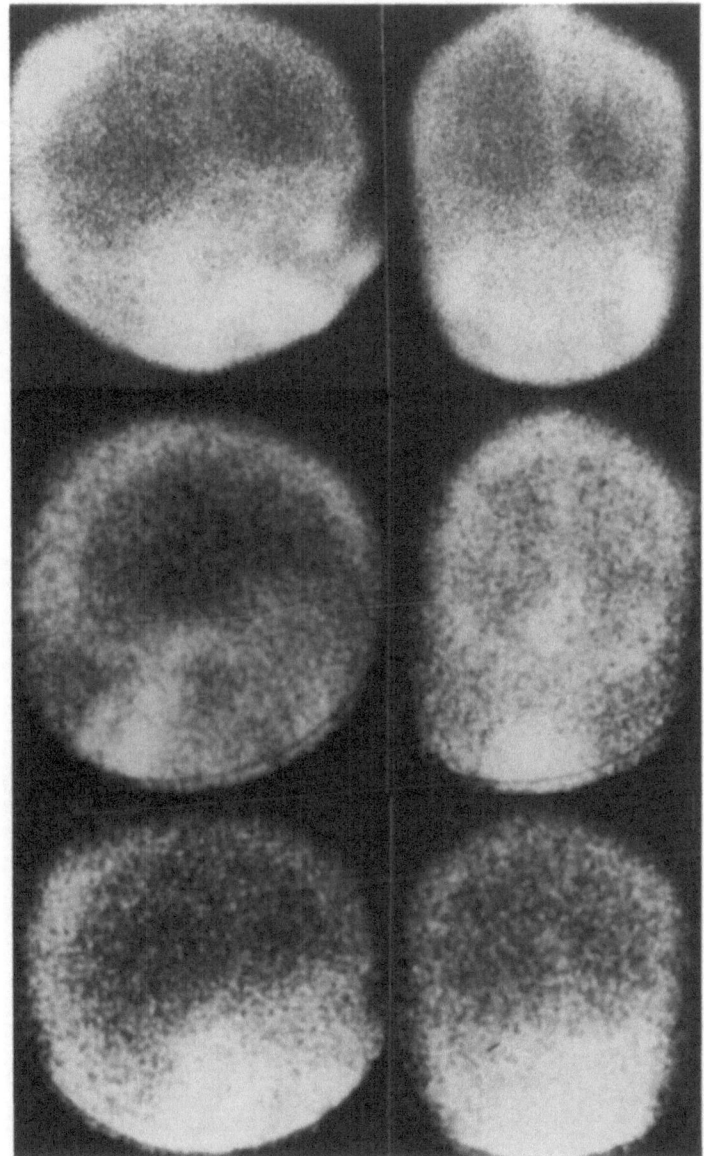

Fig. 11-13. Brain scintigraphy was performed with 99m-Tc pertechnetate (top), 99m-Tc polyphosphate (middle), and 67-Ga (below) in
a 52-year-old man with a seizure disorder who had a left temporal
lobectomy 12 years before the above studies. He is known to have
von Recklinghausen's disease. Right lateral views demonstrate
an increased amount of activity localized in the occipital area.
The abnormality is most clearly seen with 99m-Tc pertechnetate
on both the right lateral and posterior views. The site of nuclide
localization is in a neurofibroma of the scalp.

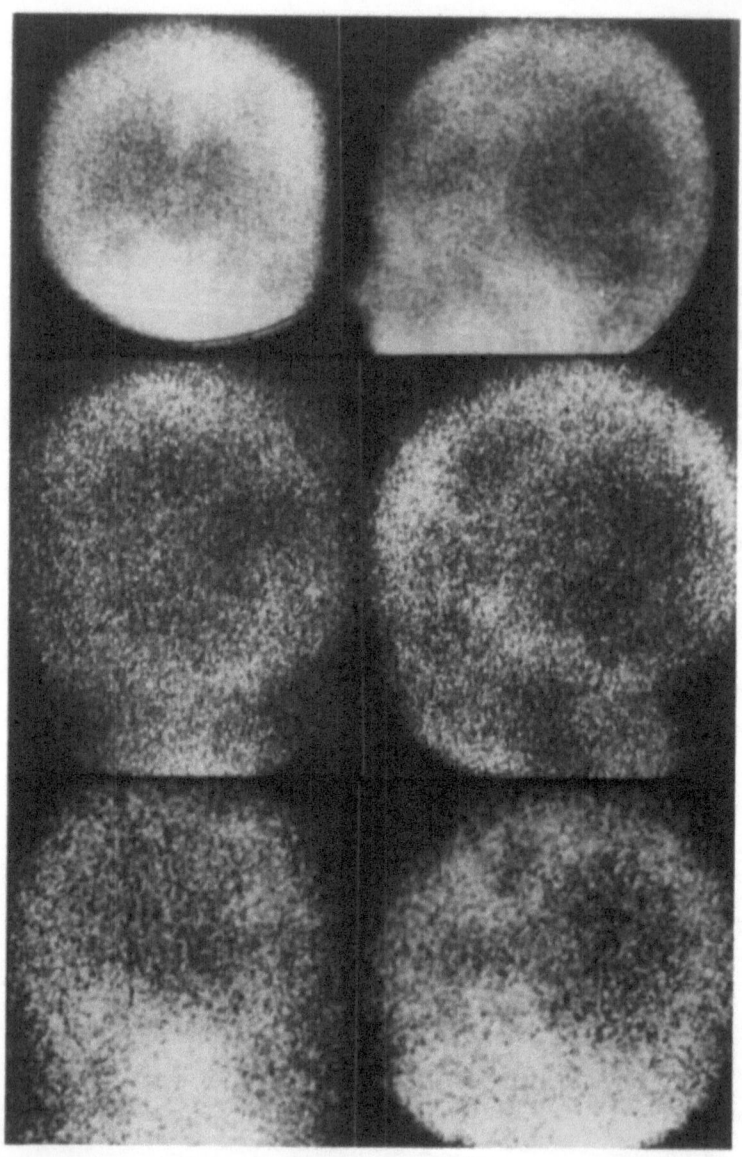

Fig. 11-14. 99m-Tc pertechnetate (top), 99m-Tc polyphosphate
(middle), and 67-Ga brain scintigraphy of a 54-year-old woman with
squamous carcinoma of the cervix, diagnosed 6 years previously.
Skull films (Fig. 11-15) revealed a lytic lesion in the area
where there is increased localization of radioactivity on the
scintigrams. Both 99m-Tc polyphosphate and 67-Ga outline the
edges of the lesion while 99m-Tc pertechnetate is more diffusely
localized in the abnormality. A subsequent excisional biopsy of
this lesion in the left parietal area showed a benign bone cyst
with fat necrosis in the center.

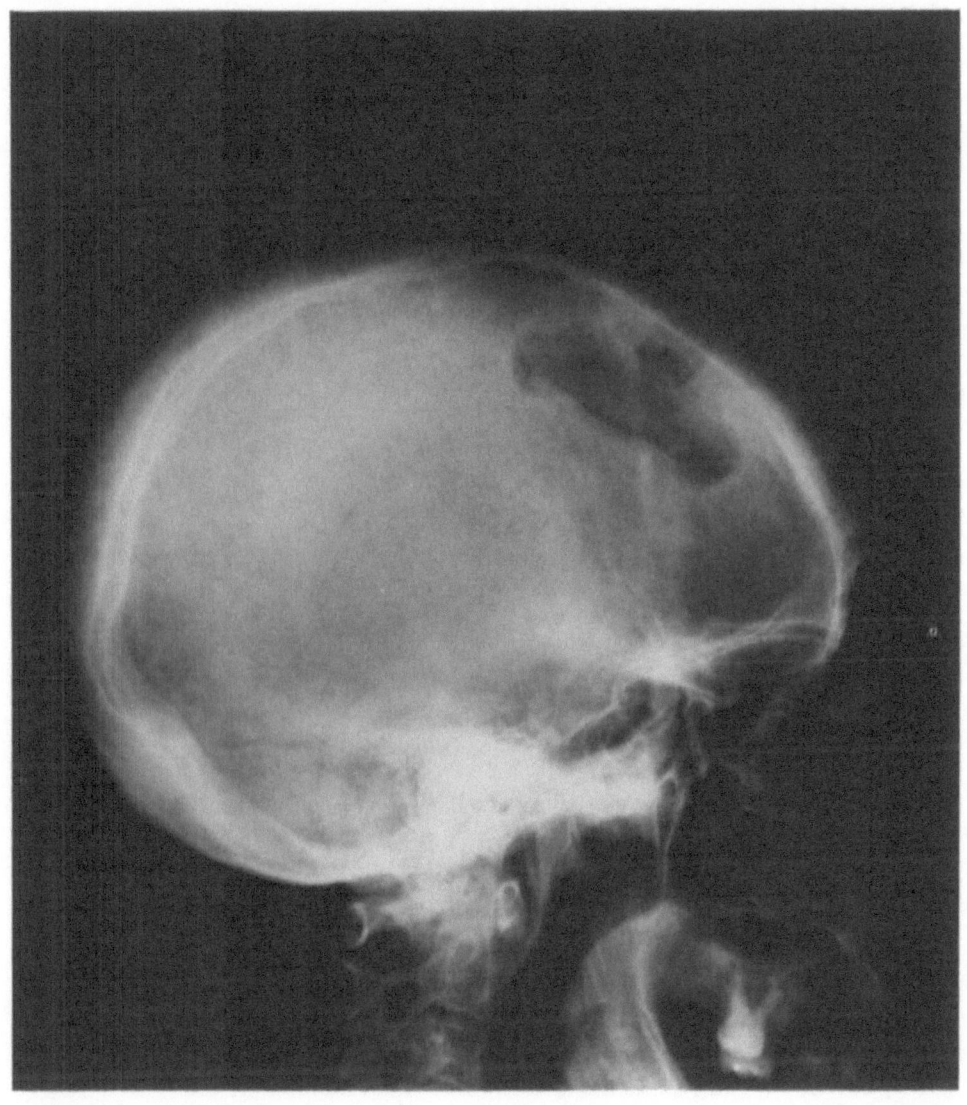

Fig. 11-15. Prebiopsy skull film of patient whose scintigrams
are shown in Fig. 11-14.

CHAPTER 12

Inflammation

Louis G. Gelrud, M. D. and Robert J. Kramer, M. D.[*]

Section on Diseases of the Liver, Metabolic Disease
    Branch, National Institute of Arthritis, Metabolism
    and Digestive Diseases

and

[*]Department of Nuclear Medicine, Clinical Center

National Institutes of Health, Bethesda, Maryland

The propensity of 67-Ga to localize within areas of inflammation was recognized during the initial investigations of the
isotope as a tumor-scanning agent (20,24,29,55). These studies
reported a number of false positive 67-Ga scans showing regions
of increased radionuclide accumulation and representing the
presence of inflammation. It was soon appreciated that the isotope
consistently localized within inflammatory lesions (21,25,32)
(Table 12-1). Consequently, the tendency for 67-Ga to concentrate
within sites of inflammation may result in a new and useful clinical test.

To date, clinical observations make up most of the information
concerning this facet of 67-Ga metabolism. A wide variety of
inflammatory lesions have been reported to concentrate 67-Ga, and
these are listed in Table I (20,24,26,27-29). Although they vary
in etiology and histology, these lesions may be visualized on 67-Ga
scan prior to the institution of appropriate therapy. After therapy
is begun, scan visualization gradually diminishes in intensity as
healing ensues (28). When healing is complete and the underlying
lesion is inactive, no visualization is observed (29).

The usefulness of 67-Ga for detecting inflammatory lesions
has been examined in a retrospective study. Of thirty patients
with acute leukemia evaluated with 67-Ga scintiscans at NIH, five

181

had clinically and histologically documented abscesses. Four of
these five patients had areas of increased localization on their
scans representative of their abscess sites. The fifth had multiple small liver abscesses which were not separable from the normal
liver uptake of 67-Ga. The site of the abscess was clinically
suspected but not documented at the time of 67-Ga scintiscanning
(33).

Recently, experimental studies have been performed to examine
67-Ga localization within inflammatory lesions (see Chapter 2).
Both deep and subcutaneous lesions were shown to be visualized by
48-72 hours after the injection of 67-Ga (32). Studies of the
acute kinetics of radionuclide localization within such abscesses
have shown that the uptake of 67-Ga by these lesions appears to
be mediated by the inflammatory granulocyte (33).

The presence of 67-Ga within inflammatory lesions is dependent
on the presence of granulocytes in the lesion. The use of 67-Ga
to detect the inflammation will produce a negative result if the
host is incapable of either producing or mobilizing granulocytes
to the site of inflammation. Experimental studies using 67-Ga
to scan abscesses in leukopenic animals has confirmed this by
showing a delay in accumulation or absence of 67-Ga at the abscess
site on scintiscan (33). Conversely, a host capable of generating
an inflammatory response to an appropriate stimulus will show
localization of 67-Ga in the inflammatory lesion on subsequent
scintigraphy. Electron microscopic autoradiography and ultracen-
trifugation studies of 67-Ga-labeled granulocytes indicate that
the binding site of 67-Ga within the granulocyte is lysosomal (23).
Thus, scanning with 67-Ga may be a useful and noninvasive method
for detecting clinically suspected or occult infection in man in
selected instances.

TABLE 12-1

INFLAMMATORY LESIONS LOCALIZING

GALLIUM-67

PULMONARY ABSCESS

ACTIVE TUBERCULOSIS

ACTIVE SARCOIDOSIS

SILICOSIS

PLEURISY

BACTERIAL PNEUMONIA

SIALADENTITIS

MYOCARDIAL INFARCT

PAGET'S DISEASE

EMPYEMA OF THE GALLBLADDER

Fig. 12-1. The patient, a 37-year-old woman
with acute myelomonocytic leukemia, developed
a painful right lower extremity over the area
of the achilles tendon which was relieved by
prednisone. When medication was discontinued,
the pain returned to the extent that she was
unable to walk. Plain x-ray films and a veno-
gram were normal. Following increased swelling
and tenderness of the site, pus was aspirated
from an abscess localized over the right
gastrocnemius muscle. A posterior 67-Ga scan
revealed an abnormal uptake of 67-Ga in the
right distal leg along the tibia and in an
area overlying the gastrocnemius muscle (arrow).
Subsequent to the 67-Ga scan, x-rays were
repeated and were interpreted as showing
tibial osteomyelitis. A calf abscess had
developed clinically.

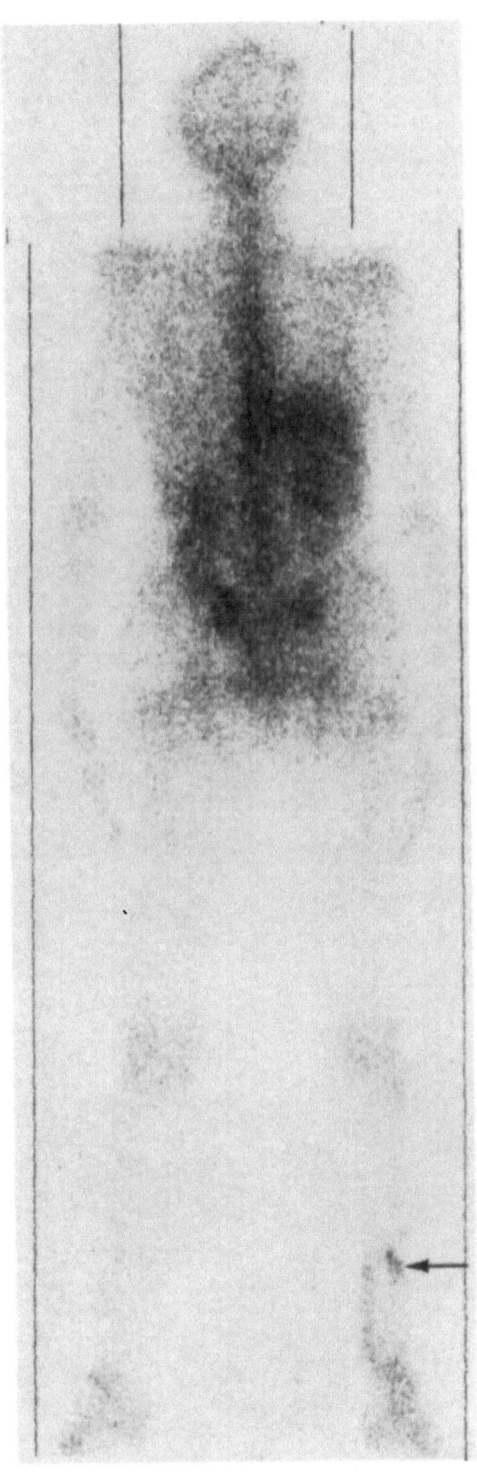

Fig. 12-2. A 56-year-old man with a
lymphocytic lymphoma underwent peritoneoscopy. Subsequently, the peritoneoscopy site became painful and erythematous
but no antibiotics were required and the
area healed uneventfully. The anterior
67-Ga scan (left) showed abnormal localization of 67-Ga at the peritoneoscopy
site. The posterior view (right) was
normal. A repeat 67-Ga scan obtained
when healing was complete showed no
abnormal accumulation of 67-Ga.

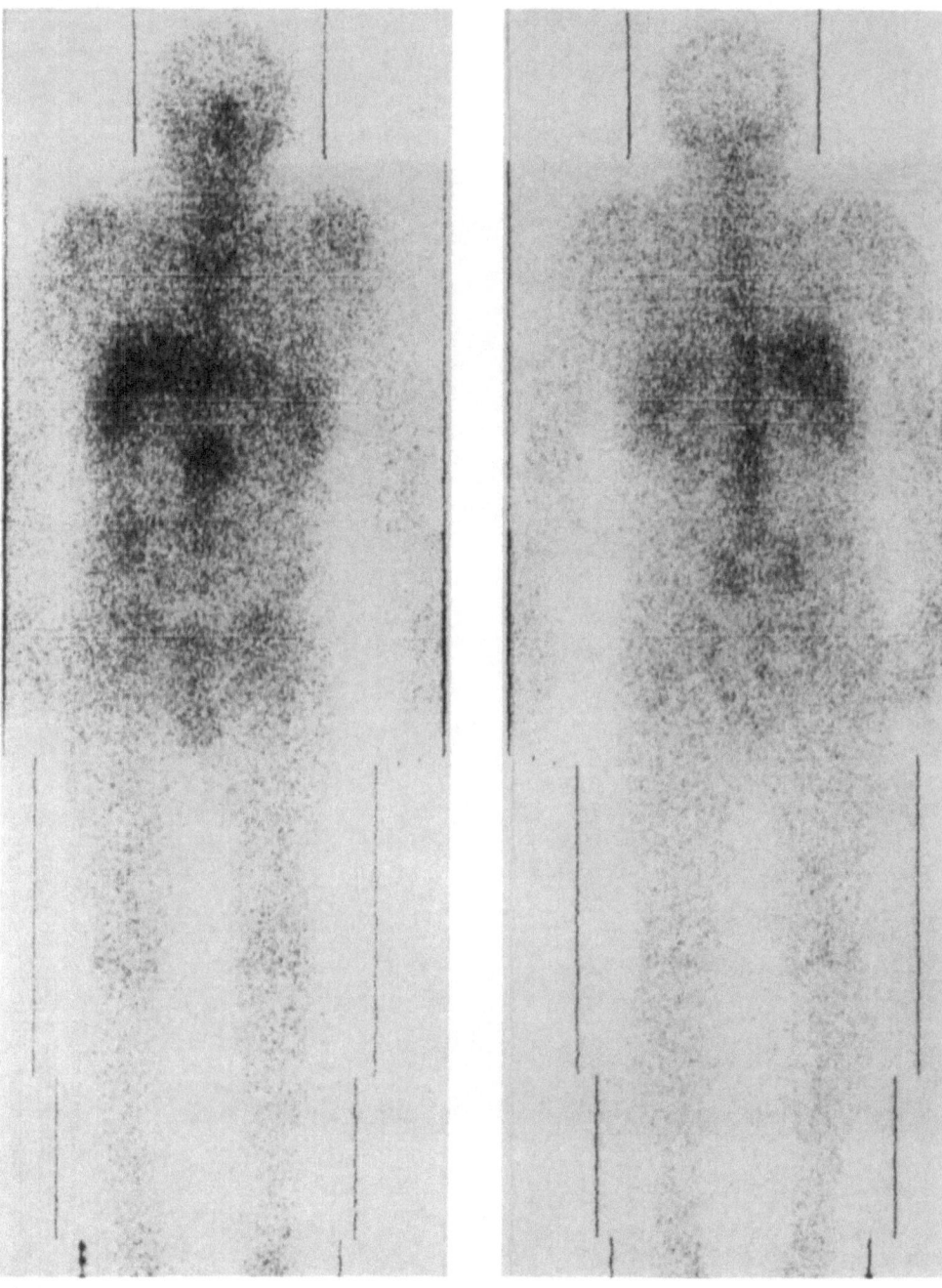

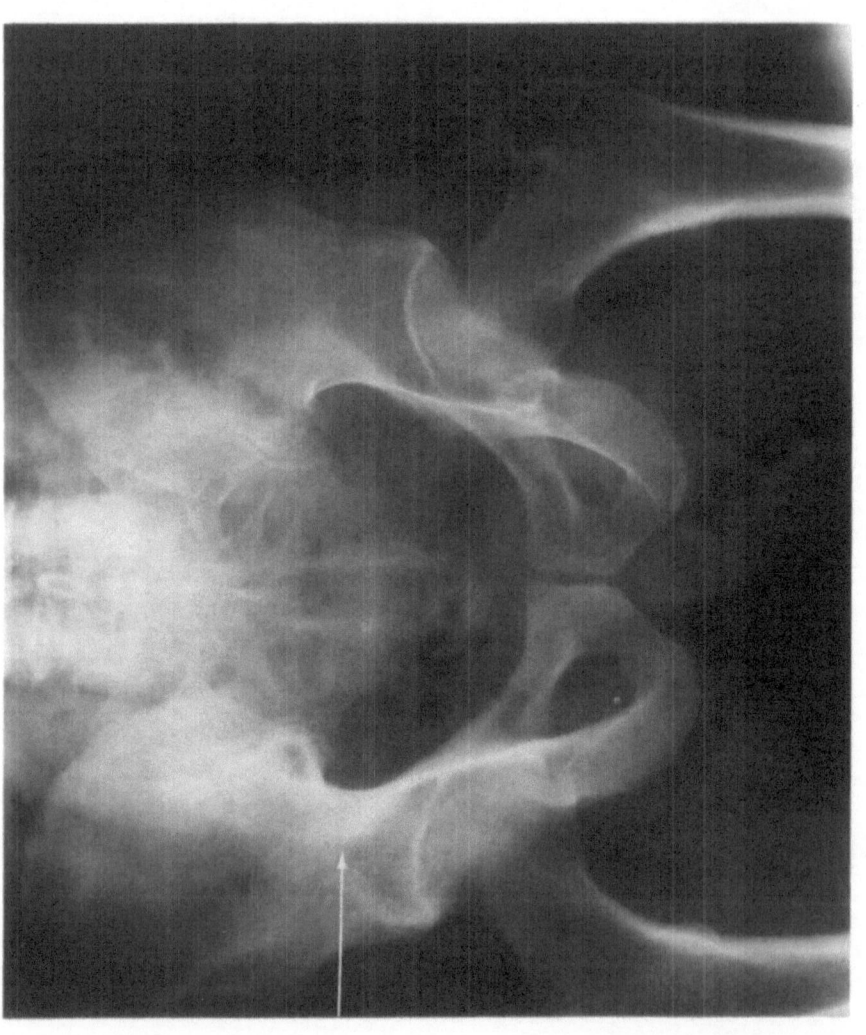

Fig. 12-3A. X-ray examination of a 59-year-old man with a histiocytic lymphoma showed a sclerotic process involving the right hemipelvis. No actual destructive foci were present and this was thought to represent Paget's disease and not lymphomatous spread.

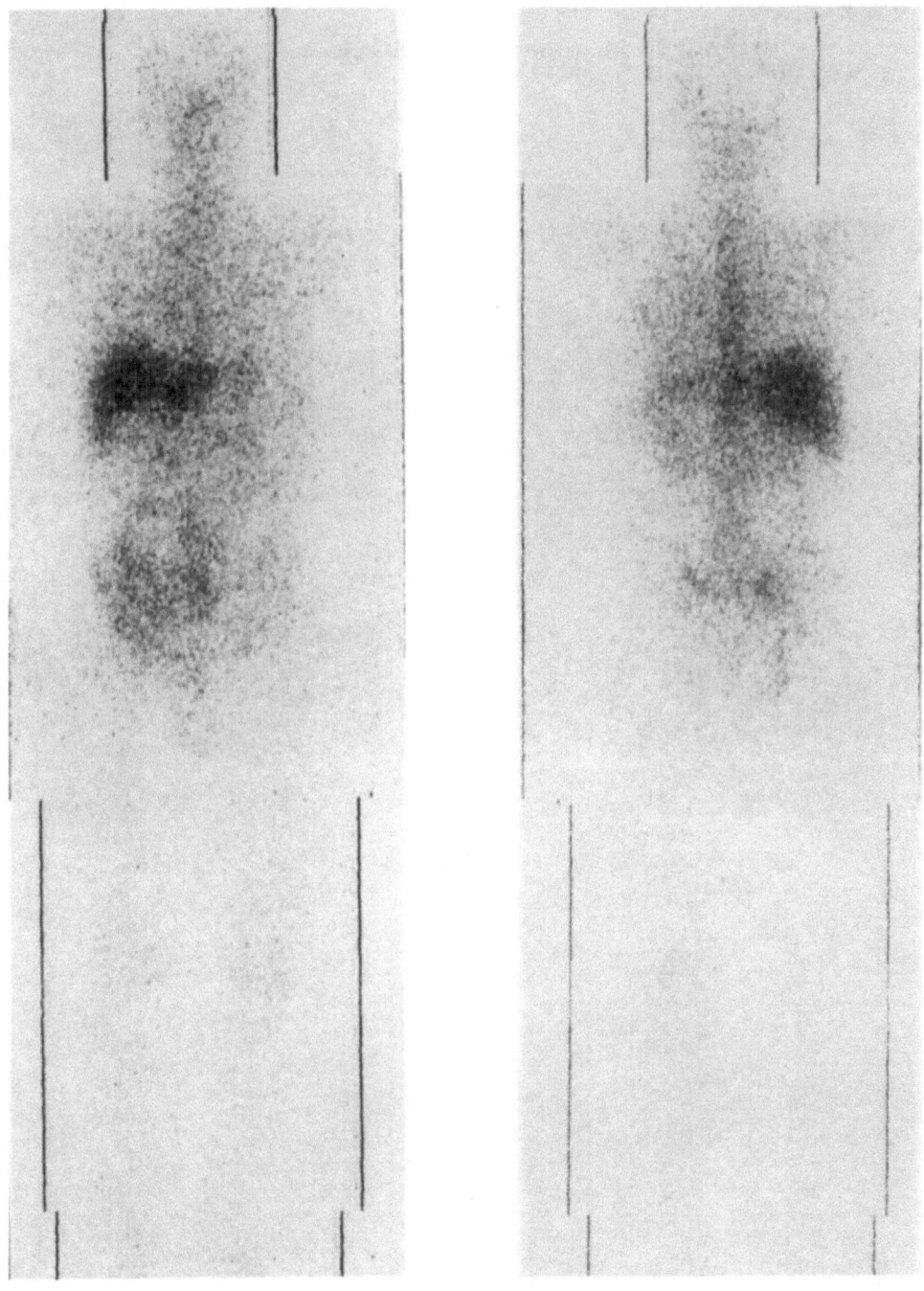

Fig. 12-3B. Increased accumulation of 67-Ga throughout the right side of the pelvis was present on the anterior and posterior 67-Ga scans.

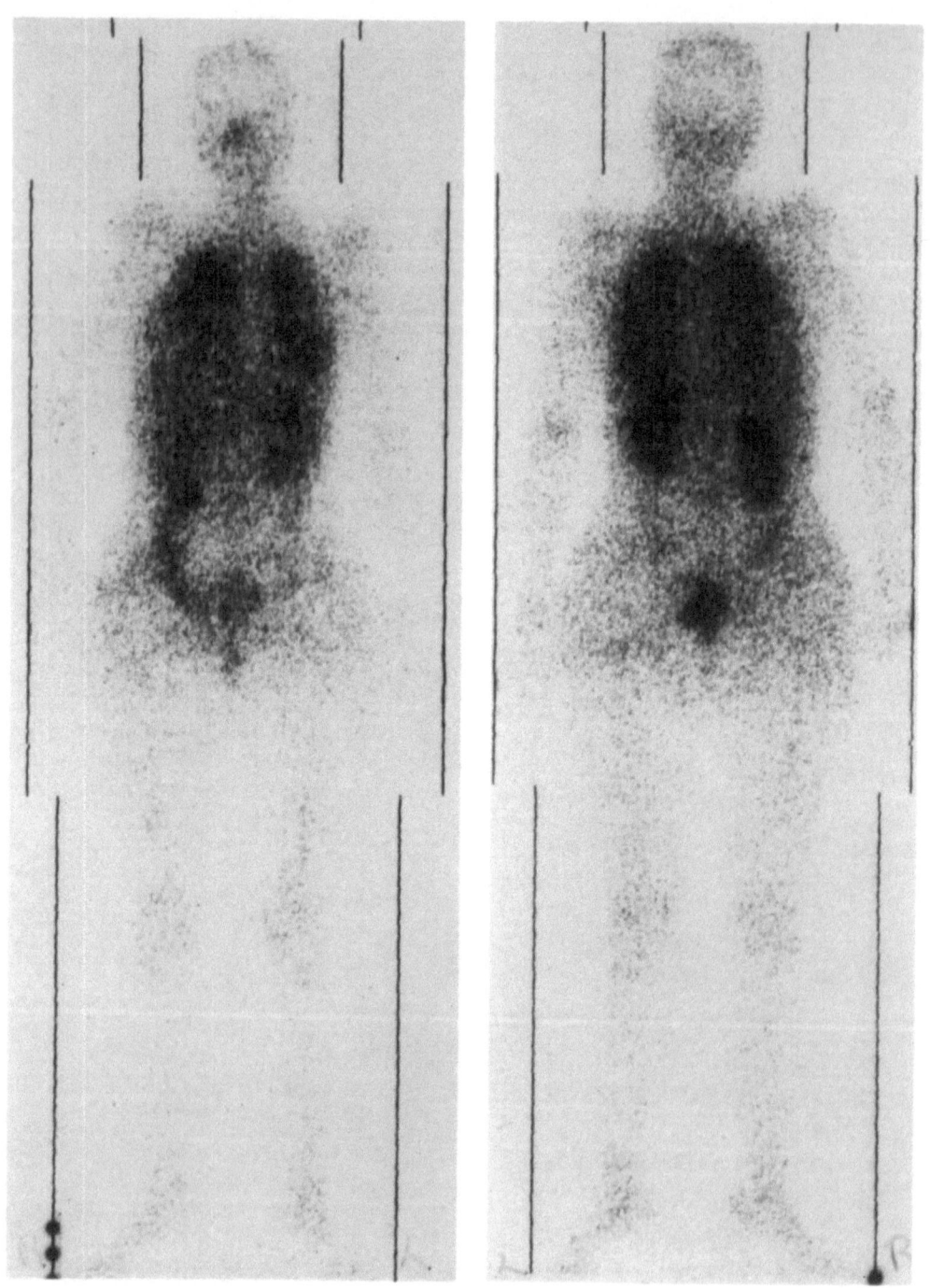

Fig. 12-4. A 32-year-old woman with
biopsy proven stage III-A Hodgkin's
disease developed fatigue, shortness
of breath, dyspnea on exertion, anorexia, and weakness. Diffuse inter-
stitial and alveolar infiltrates were
seen bilaterally on the chest radiograph. Percutaneous lung biopsy
recovered Pneumocystis carinii.
Significant colonies of E. coli grew
on urine cultures and three blood
cultures were positive with the same
organism. The patient recovered
uneventfully on antibiotic therapy.
Diffuse abnormal accumulations of 67-Ga
were present throughout both lungs and
both kidneys on anterior and posterior
scans. This was interpreted as
representing bilateral pneumonitis
and pyelonephritis. Subsequent to
therapy, repeat 67-Ga scans were
normal.

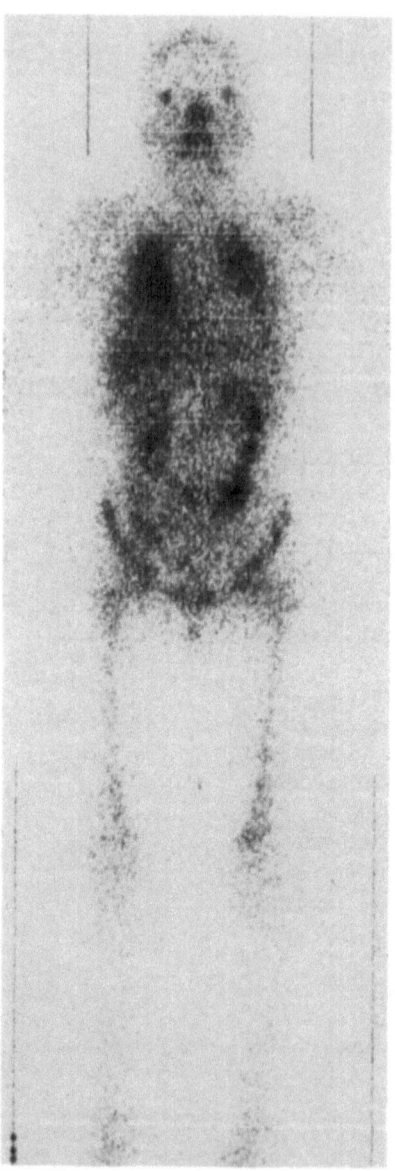 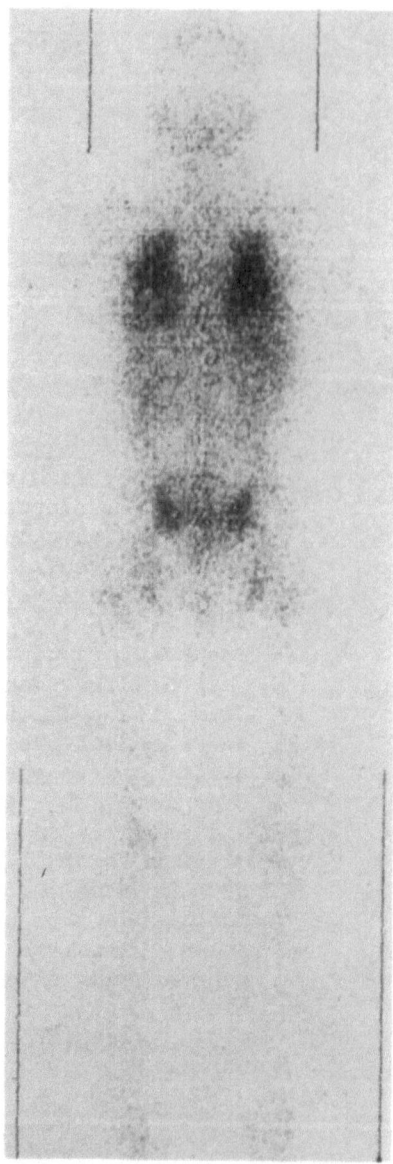

Fig. 12-5. A 25-year-old woman with treated Hodgkin's disease
noted the onset of intermittent low-grade fever and a moderate,
nonproductive cough approximately 9 months after cessation of
therapy. Roentgenographically, she had bilateral pneumonitis.
This stabilized over a several-day-period without treatment and
gradually resulted in moderate fibrotic changes on x-ray with
complete resolution of symptoms. Scans reveal accumulation of
67-Ga in both lung fields. A repeat 67-Ga scan, 6 months later,
did not show abnormal pulmonary deposition of 67-Ga.

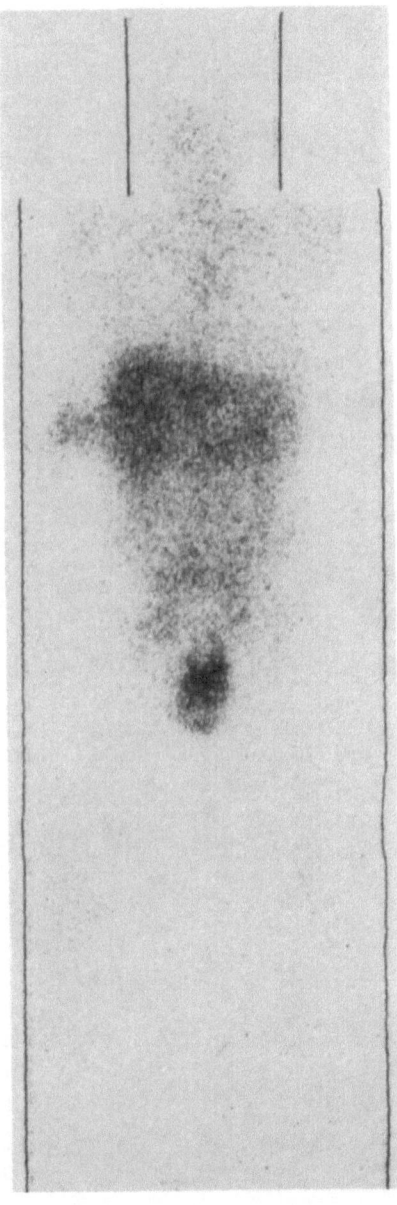

Fig. 12-6. A 29-year-old man with acute myelocytic leukemia developed a scrotal abscess during initial therapy. The abscess did not respond to the usual treatment including antibiotics. Intensive local and antibiotic therapy was then instituted in addition to antileukemic chemotherapy with healing of the abscess. The 67-Ga scan was obtained when therapy was initiated and it revealed marked localization of 67-Ga in the area of the scrotum. (Injection site is seen in right arm.)

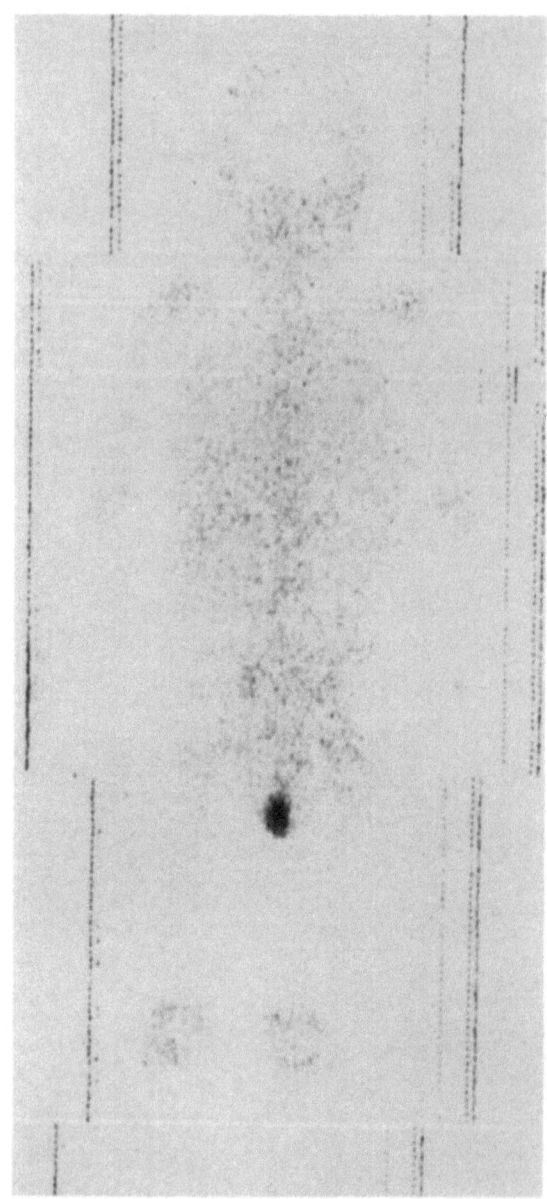

Fig. 12-7. A 5-year-old boy with a two-year history of acute
lymphocytic leukemia was being treated intrathecally for meningeal
involvement. At the time of the scan he was leukopenic from his
medication and had developed vomiting, diarrhea, and extreme
lethargy secondary to septic shock. A rectal abscess was diagnosed
and subsequently drained. The anterior 67-Ga scan, obtained prior
to draining of the abscess, revealed an abnormal accumulation of
67-Ga in the area of the rectum.

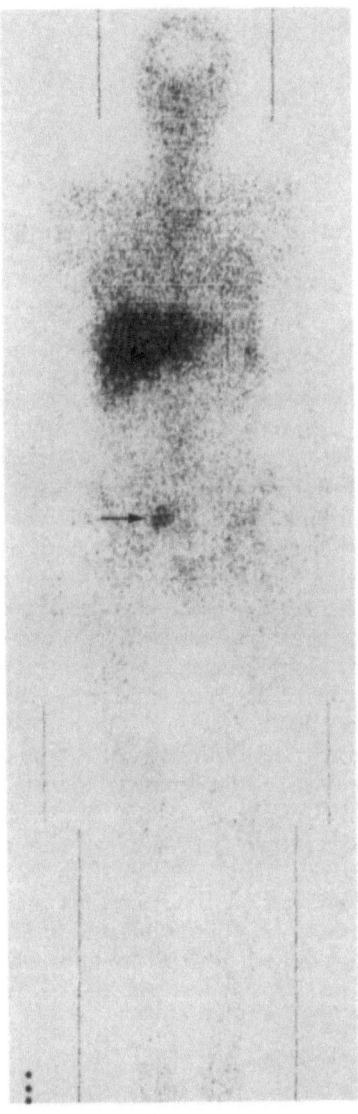

Fig. 12-8. The patient, a 43-year-old woman, had dilitation and
curettage and biopsy of her uterine cervix which showed squamous
cell carcinoma, clinically staged as 1B. Postoperatively she
developed peritonitis and a tender right adnexal mass. Antibiotic
therapy was followed by resolution of her peritonitis but not the
adnexal mass. A radical hysterectomy was advised for therapy of
her neoplasm. A biopsy of the adnexal mass showed it to be a
chronic periovarian abscess. The anterior 67-Ga scan obtained
prior to hysterectomy reveals an abnormal accumulation of 67-Ga
in the right pelvic region believed to represent the pelvic abscess.
Note 67-Ga localization in both breasts.

Fig. 12-9. A 14-year-old boy with acute
myelogenous leukemia was admitted to the
hospital with leukopenia, neutropenia with
peripheral blast forms, thrombocytopenia
and continuing high fever despite the
empirical administration of antibiotic
therapy. Multiple cultures were normal.
Left axillary adenitis was diagnosed,
aspirated, cultured and grew Pseudomonas
aeruginosa. Appropriate therapy was begun
and the patient became afebrile and the
lesion resolved. An anterior 67-Ga scan
obtained prior to discovery of the axillary
adenitis revealed abnormal accumulation of
67-Ga in the region of the left axilla.
The accumulation of 67-Ga in the right
upper abdominal and right lower chest
region represents liver activity. The
increased activity noted in both kidneys
was not suspected prior to scanning. This
was shown to represent leukemic infiltration of these organs.

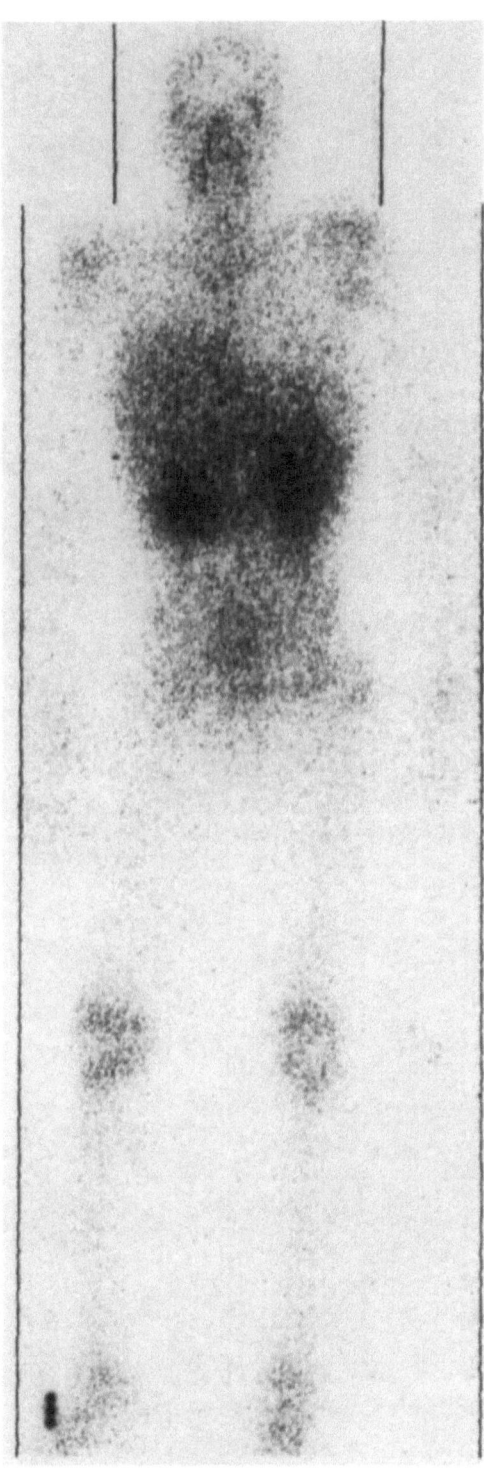

CHAPTER 13

Clinical Applications

Robert J. Kramer, M. D.

Department of Nuclear Medicine, Clinical Center

National Institutes of Health, Bethesda, Maryland

The soft-tissue affinity of radiopharmaceutical 67-Ga has widespread clinical use in the localization of sites of neoplastic disease and inflammation. However, the ultimate place of this technique in the medical armamentarium is not fully established. Despite this fact, several areas of clinical usefulness have begun to emerge.

We believe that the clinical indications for 67-Ga scans are presently: (1) suspected neoplastic disease, (2) determining extent of involvement with malignancy (staging), (3) follow-up of tumor therapy and screening for tumor recurrences, and (4) evaluation of fever of unknown origin. The use of the 67-Ga scan as a supplement to standard radiographic and laboratory procedures will be discussed below.

Screening Procedure: Because of its ease of performance and low risk to the patient, the 67-Ga scan may be of value as a screening test for malignancy or occult inflammatory disease.

Value in Detection of Unsuspected Neoplastic Lesions: Review of the first 250 cases investigated with 67-Ga citrate at the National Institutes of Health revealed positive studies in 13 cases with neoplastic disease at the time that clinical and radiographic evaluation revealed no evidence of involvement at these sites (64). While this is a small patient series, it represents a highly selected group in a referral hospital. Presumably the use of the 67-Ga scan as a screening test would have a much greater yield in detecting unknown lesions. Nonetheless, the 67-Ga scan findings offered an independent contribution to the evaluation of neoplasms by localizing optimum biopsy sites and influencing medical management in several cases.

Abnormalities on the 67-Ga scan, that were the first evidence of disease, occurred at a variety of sites (Table 1-13). The scan was most helpful in detecting mediastinal, intra-abdominal or retroperitoneal tumor and lymph node metastases.

Aid in Studying Effectiveness of Treatment: Recent studies have shown evidence of differential 67-Ga accumulation in treated and untreated patients with neoplastic disease. In a series of 120 patients reported by Langhammer (24), all 78 patients with untreated tumors were positive on 67-Ga scan. Of the 42 patients with neoplasms treated with radiation or chemotherapy, 25 were negative at the time of scan and 17 were positive.

There is, as yet, no information on the survival in treated cases with negative scans compared with those with positive studies; nor are there any studies correlating the ability of neoplastic tissue to concentrate 67-Ga with its malignant potential. While this association is not definitely proven, the occurrence of a negative 67-Ga scan following tumor therapy is consistent with effective treatment whereas a positive study is evidence for recurrent disease or inadequate therapy.

The value of the 67-Ga scan in serially following the effect of tumor therapy and in screening for recurrences may be seen in the subsequent case records.

It is evident, from the material presented, that 67-Ga is capable of localizing in a wide spectrum of neoplastic and inflammatory diseases. As with other techniques in nuclear medicine, 67-Ga scanning is a noninvasive procedure. It lends itself easily to serial studies involving initial diagnosis, staging, and effect of therapy in patients with occult infections and neoplastic disease.

TABLE 13-1

67-Ga Uptake in 13 Patients with
Unsuspected Sites of Neoplastic Disease

Site	No.
Lymph Node Groups	3
Mediastinum and Hilar Areas	3
Intra-abdominal and Retroperitoneal Lesions	5
Lung	1
Skeleton, Bone Marrow	2
Liver	3

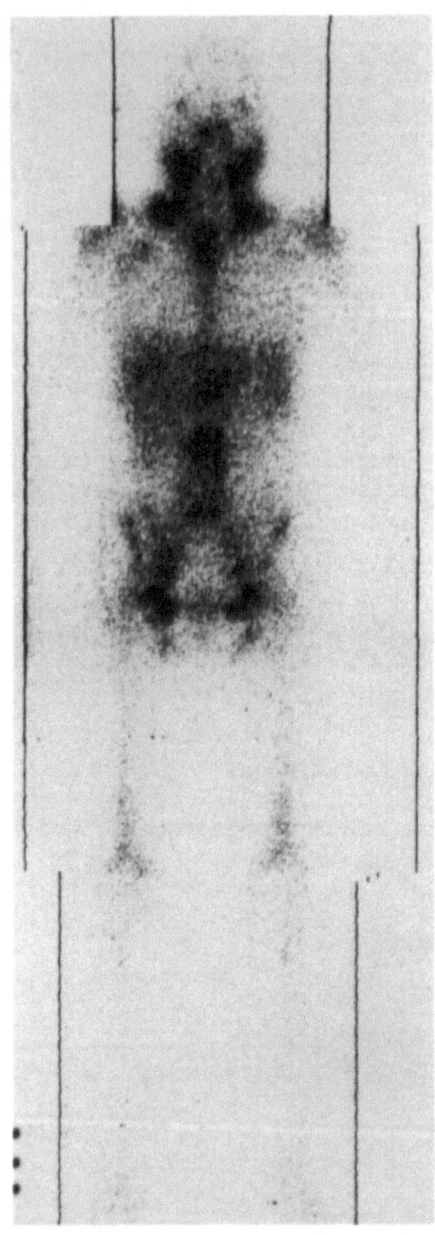

Fig. 13-1A. Anterior 67-Ga scan of a 45-year-old woman with a
histiocytic lymphoma. The initial study reveals prominent uptake
in the cervical, supraclavicular, and axillary lymph node chains
bilaterally; and the mediastinum, retroperitoneal, paraaortic,
and ilio-inguinal node groups. In addition, there is evidence
of marrow expansion with isotope uptake in the distal portions
of the femurs.

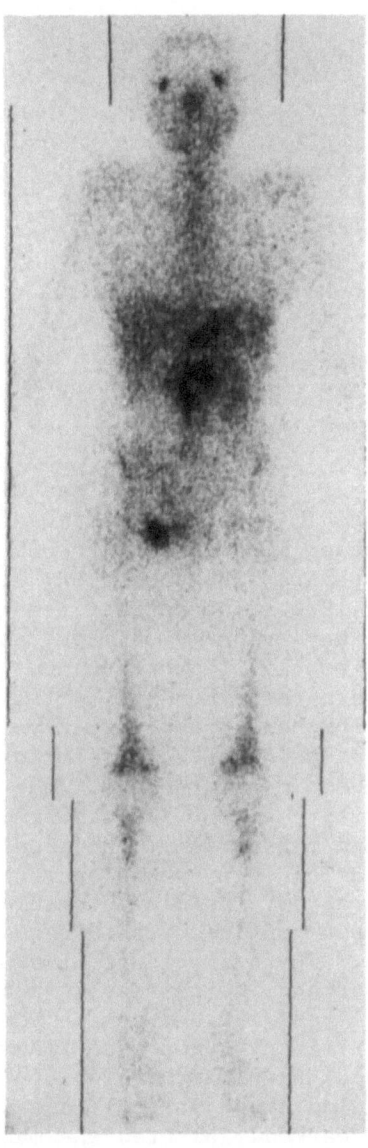

Fig. 13-1B. A repeat scan was performed 8 months later when the patient returned complaining of abdominal pain. Clinically, the only known area of residual disease was in the right inguinal region. The patient had received both radiation and chemotherapy. This second scan reveals persistent nuclide concentration in the previously noted abdominal site. The right inguinal area is also positive. The marrow uptake is more extensive than noted on the earlier study with additional localization of 67-Ga in the proximal tibias bilaterally probably representing expanded marrow consistent with antitumor therapy or neoplastic involvement.

Fig. 13-2. A 27-year-old man with previously
diagnosed II-A Hodgkin's disease received
total nodal irradiation of 4000 rads to
all lymph node areas between July 1969 and
January 1970. The patient remained well,
without any evidence of recurrent disease,
until March 1972, when routine chest x-rays
revealed a recurrent mediastinal mass.
Repeat lymphangiography, x-rays, and bone
marrow biopsies of both anterior iliac
crests were nondiagnostic. The 67-Ga scan
was positive at the left anterior iliac
crest and mediastinum. Because of the iliac
crest lesions, an open biopsy was performed
in this area. Histologic sections of the
left crest confirmed the diagnosis of Hodgkin's
disease. In this patient, the 67-Ga scan
was important in the staging procedure. The
patient's stage was changed from II to IV as
a result of the 67-Ga scan finding and the
consequent open marrow biopsy. No other
studies indicated stage IV disease. This
finding markedly altered the management of
the patient.

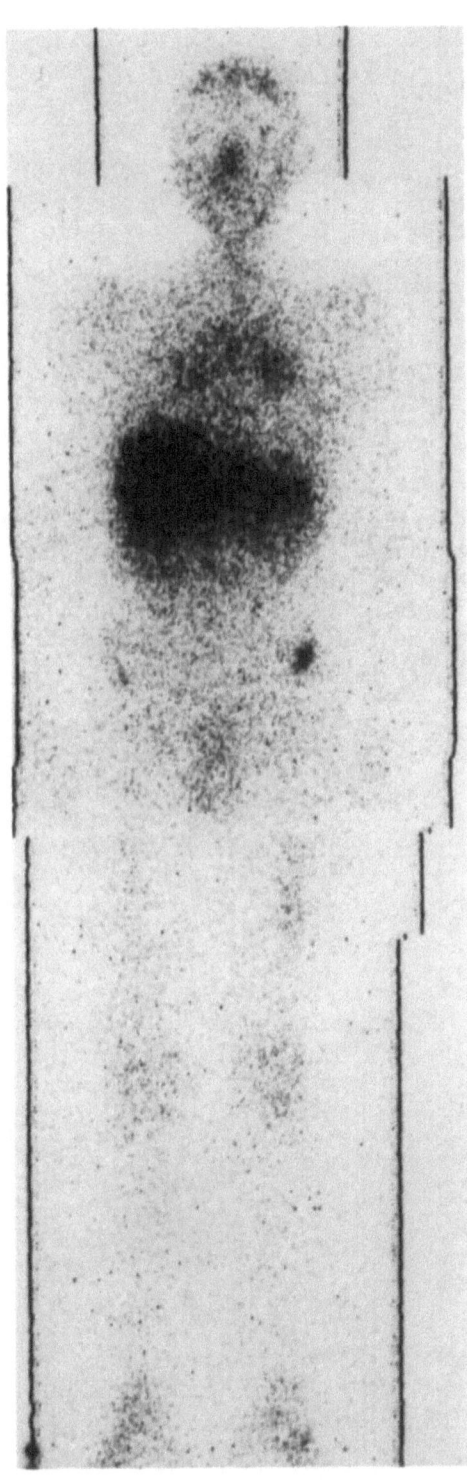

Fig. 13-3. Anterior 67-Ga scan of a
52-year-old man with a hepatoma of the
right hepatic lobe. The 67-Ga scan
reveals homogeneous uptake throughout
the liver. There is a distant metastasis to the right cervical chain
which was not clinically detected.

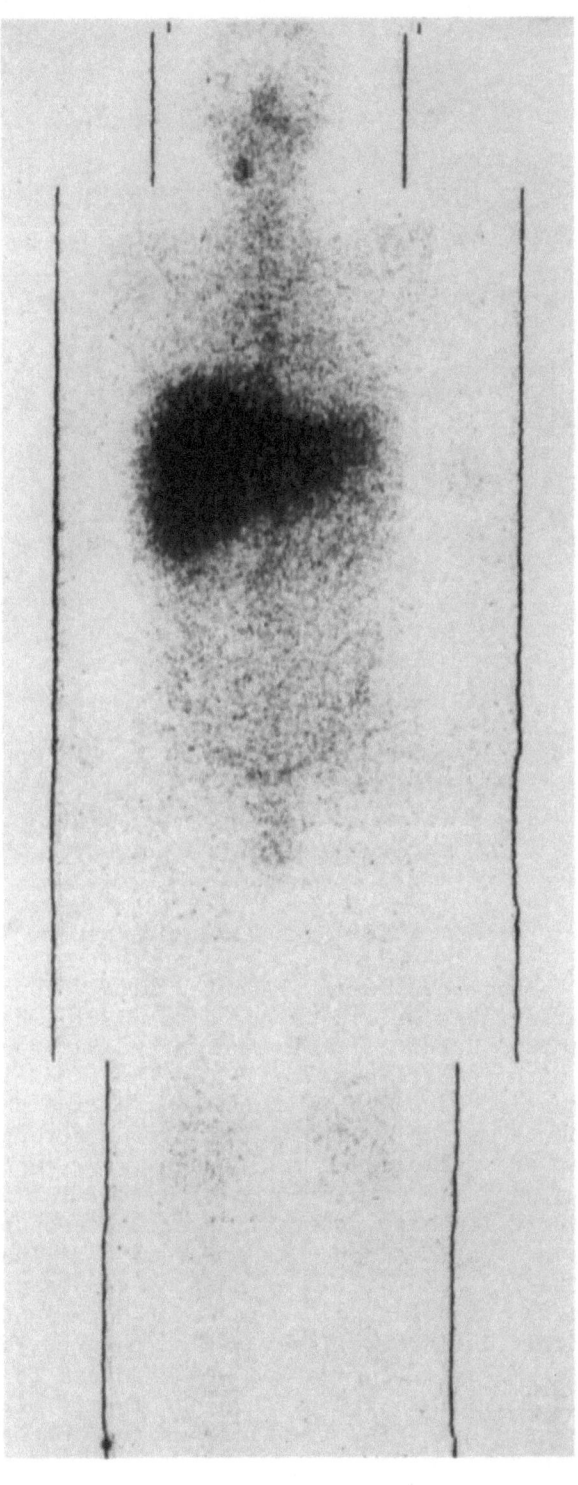

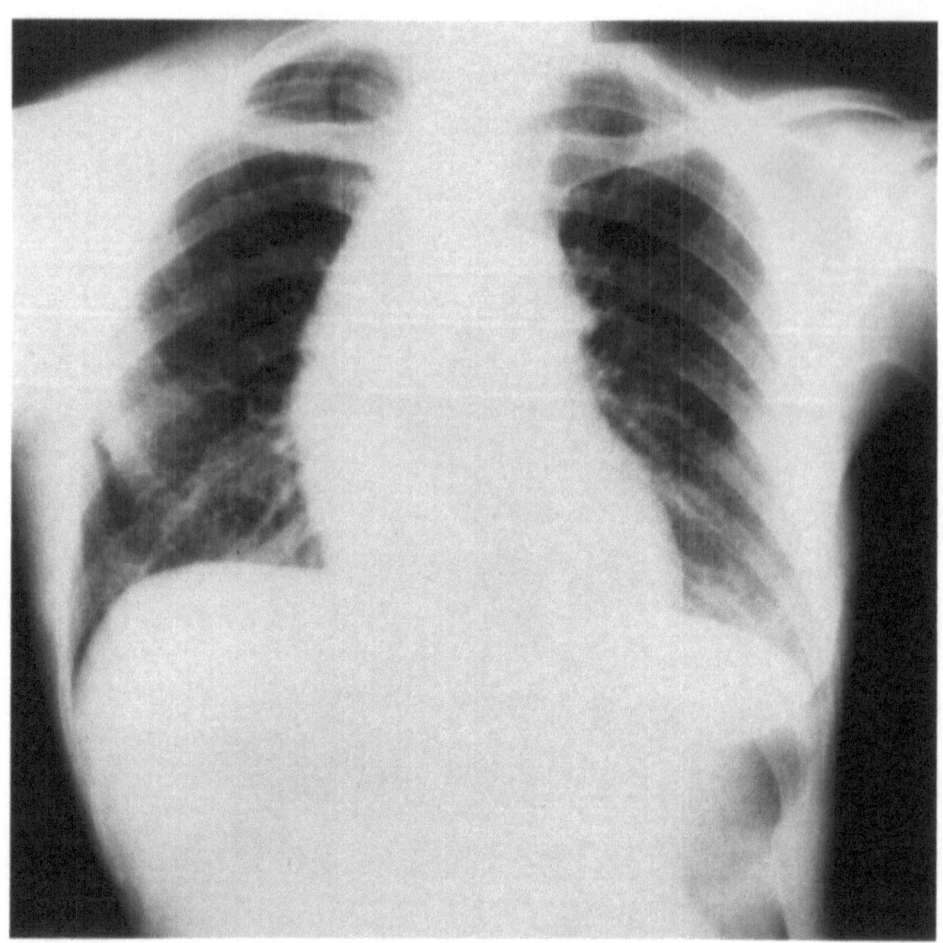

Fig. 13-4A. A 45-year-old woman presented with a fever of unknown
origin. The patient was well until December 1971, when she was
found to be anemic. Hospitalization in March 1972 documented a
febrile course with temperatures to 39°C without chills or sweats.
Laboratory evaluation revealed an elevated alkaline phosphatase.
A liver scan showed multiple defects. A second strength PPD was
positive. Chest and gallbladder radiographs, IVP, upper GI series,
and barium enema were all within normal limits. The patient underwent an exploratory laparotomy revealing aortic adenopathy and
multiple discrete liver lesions. A biopsy of the liver on frozen
section was initially interpreted as showing neoplasm. Consequently, an aortic dissection was not performed. Permanent histologic
sections demonstrated fibrous tissue but no tumor. The patient
continued to run a febrile course and was referred to the NIH.
Initial physical examination revealed hepatomegaly with no lymph-
adenopathy. Chest x-ray (Fig. 13-4A) shows thoracic scoliosis with
no definite mediastinal mass.

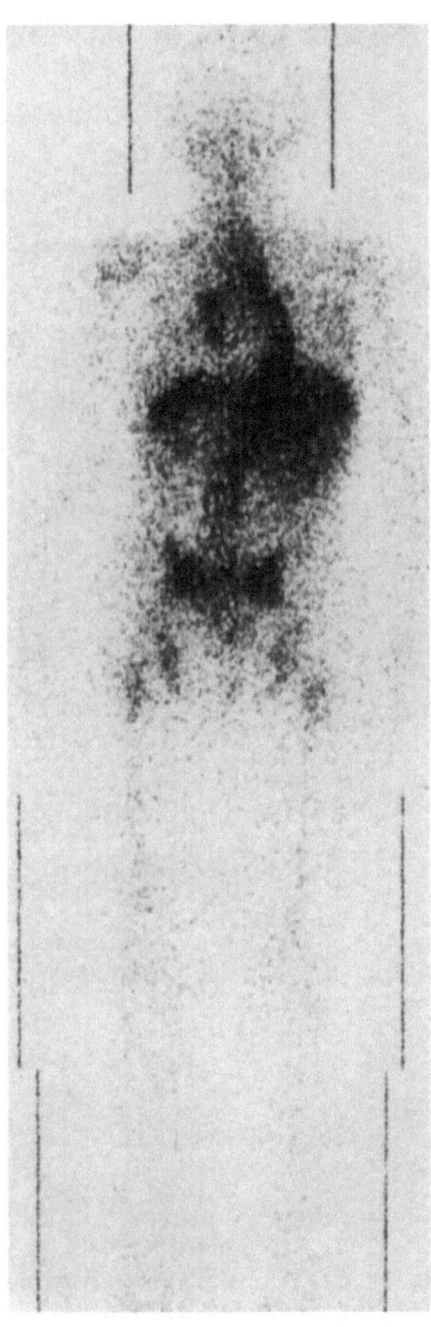

Fig. 13-4B.   67-Ga scan demonstrates mediastinal and left hilar
masses.   Tomograms of the mediastinum were subsequently performed,
revealing left hilar adenopathy.   Repeat exploratory laparotomy
with node biopsy demonstrated Hodgkin's disease.

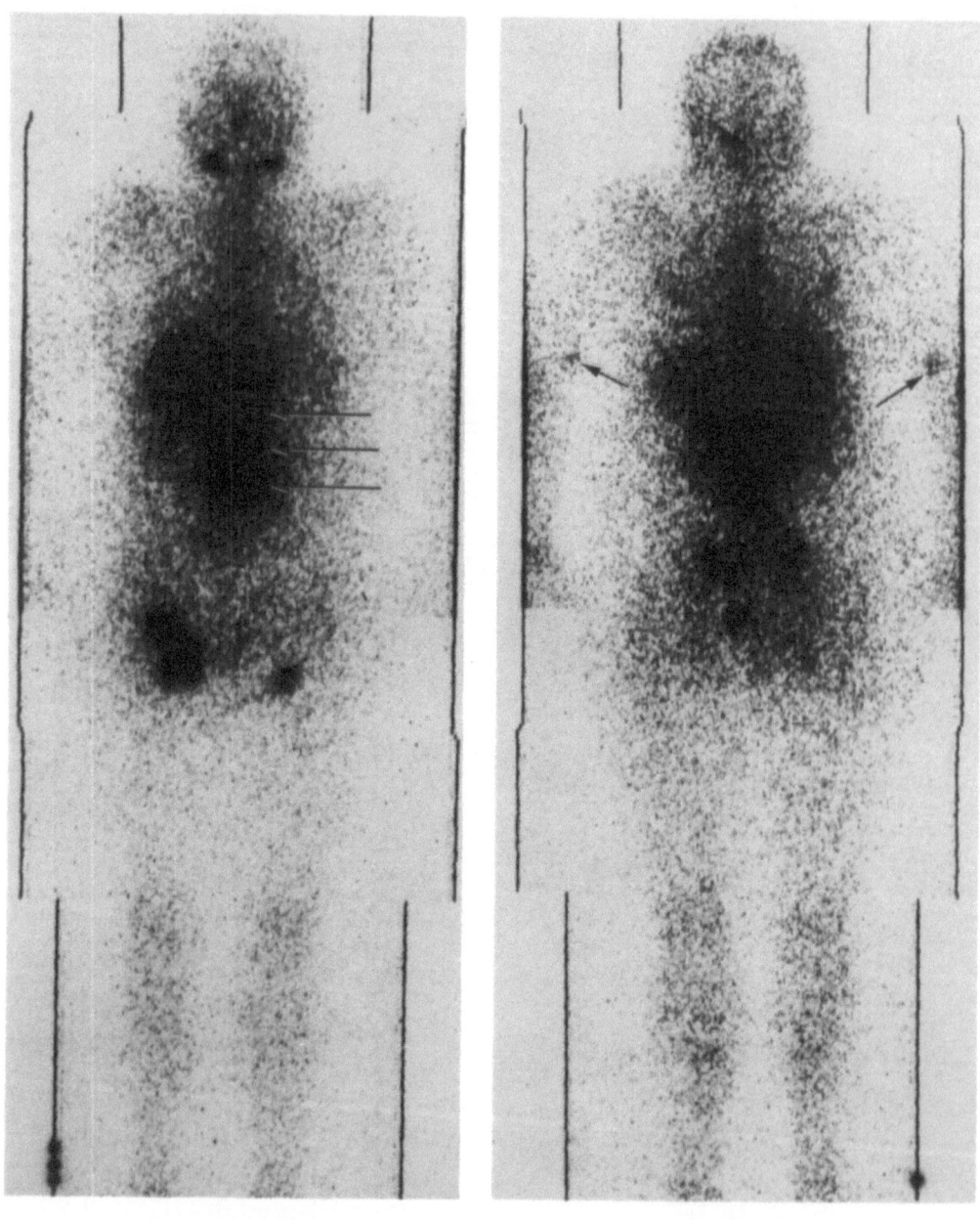

Fig. 13-5A.   67-Ga scan of a 52-year-old woman with histiocytic
lymphoma.   Initial staging revealed ilioinguinal, axillary and
submandibular involvement.   Lymphangiogram was inadequate with no
ascent of dye above L-2.   Anterior 67-Ga scan reveals an unsuspected
abdominal mass, in addition to the clinically known inguinal and
submandibular regions.   The posterior 67-Ga scan demonstrates
bilateral epitrochlear nodes.

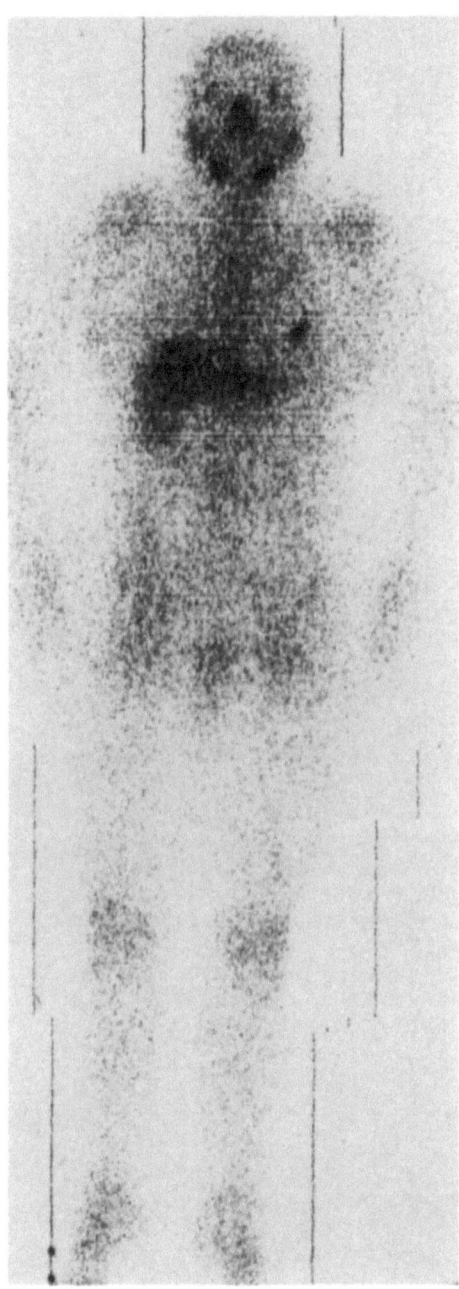

Fig. 13-5B. Following radiation and chemotherapy, a repeat anterior 67-Ga scan 6 months later reveals residual uptake in the submandibular glands. The previously noted epigastric mass and ilioinguinal nodes have resolved; however, there is a new lesion in the left anterior rib cage.

REFERENCES

1. Dudley, H.C., Maddox, G.E., LaRue, H.C. Studies of the metabolism of gallium. J Pharmacol Exp Ther 96: 135-138, 1949.

2. Dudley, H.C., Maddox, G.E. Deposition of radio gallium (Ga^{72}) in skeletal tissues. J Pharmacol Exp Ther 96: 224-227, 1949.

3. Dudley, H.C., Imirie, G.W., Istock, J.T. Deposition of radiogallium (Ga^{72}) in proliferating tissues. Radiology 55: 571-578, 1950.

4. Mulry, W.C., Dudley, H.C. Studies of radiogallium as a diagnostic agent in bone tumors. J Lab Clin Med 37: 239-252, 1951.

5. King, E.R., Brady, L.W., Dudley, H.C. Therapeutic trials of radiogallium (Ga^{72}). A report of four cases. Arch Intern Med 90: 785-789, 1952.

6. Bruner, H.D., Hayes, R.L., Perkinson, J.D. A study of gallium^{72}. Preliminary data on gallium 67. Radiology 61: 602-612, 1953.

7. Hayes, R.L., Carlton, J.E., Byrd, B.L. Bone scanning with gallium-68: a carrier effect. J Nucl Med 6: 605-610, 1965.

8. Gynning, I., Langeland, P., Lindberg, S., Waldeskog, B. Localization with Sr^{85} of spinal metastases in mammary cancer and changes in uptake after hormone and roentgen therapy. A preliminary report. Acta Radiol 55: 119-128, 1961.

9. Blau, M., Nagler, W., Bender, M.A. Fluorine-18: a new isotope for bone scanning. J Nucl Med 3: 332-334, 1962.

10. Edwards, C.L., Hayes, R.L. Tumor scanning with ^{67}Ga citrate. Preliminary note. J Nucl Med 10: 103-105, 1969.

11. Lewis, J.E. The radiochemistry of aluminum and gallium. Washington, Subcommittee on Radiochemistry, National Academy of Sciences, National Research Council, 1961.

12. Dudley, H.C. Gallium citrate and radio-gallium (Ga^{72}) citrate.
    J Am Chem Soc 72: 3822-3823, 1950.

13. Hayes, R.L., Edwards, C.L. New applications of tumor-localizing
    radiopharmaceuticals. Proceedings of the International Atomic
    Energy Agency Symposium on Medical Radioisotope Scintigraphy.
    Monte Carlo, Principality of Monaco, October 23-28, 1972. In
    press.

14. Milder, M.S., Frankel, R.S., Bulkley, G.B., Ketcham, A.S.,
    Johnston, G.S. Gallium-67 scintigraphy in malignant melanoma.
    Cancer. In press.

15. Arseneau, J.C., Sponzo, R.W., Aamodt, R.L., Evans, W.,
    Johnston, G.S., Canellos, G.P. Granulocytic incorporation of
    67-gallium in human bone marrow and peripheral blood.
    Submitted, 1972 Annual Meeting of the American Society of
    Hematology.

16. Nelson, B., Hayes, R.L., Edwards, C.L., Kniseley, R.M.,
    Andrews, G.A. Distribution of gallium in human tissues after
    intravenous administration. J Nucl Med 13: 92-100, 1972.

17. Larson, S.M., Milder, M.S., Johnston, G.S. Interpretation of
    the ^{67}Ga photoscan. J Nucl Med 14: 208-214, 1973.

18. Edwards, C.L., Hayes, R.L. Scanning malignant neoplasms with
    gallium 67. JAMA 212: 1182-1190, 1970.

19. Vaidya, S.G., Chaudhri, M.A., Morrison, R., Whait, D.
    Localisation of gallium-67 in malignant neoplasms. Lancet 2:
    911-914, 1970.

20. Higasi, T., Nakayama, Y., Murata, A., Nakamura, K., Sugiyama,
    M., Kawaguchi, T., Suzuki, S. Clinical evaluation of ^{67}Ga-
    citrate scanning. J Nucl Med 13: 196-201, 1972.

21. Gelrud, L.G., Arseneau, J.C., Johnston, G.S. Gallium-67
    localization in experimental and clinical abscesses. Clin
    Res 21: 600, 1973.

22. Brown, D.H., Swartzendruber, D.C., Carlton, J.E., Byrd, B.L.,
    Hayes, R.L. Mechanism of gallium-binding in tumors: isolation
    and characterization of gallium binding-granules (GBG) in
    soft tissue tumors. Proc Amer Assoc Cancer Res 13: 37, 1972.

23. Swartzendruber, D.C., Nelson, B., Hayes, R.L. Gallium-67
    localization in lysosomal-like granules of leukemic and non-
    leukemic murine tissues. J Natl Cancer Inst 46: 941-952,
    1971.

24. Langhammer, H., Glaubitt, G., Grebe, S.F., Hampe, J.F., Haubold, U., Hör, G., Kaul, A., Koeppe, P., Koppenhagen, J., Roedler, H.D., van der Schoot, J.B. ^{67}Ga for tumor scanning. J Nucl Med 13: 25-30, 1972.

25. Ito, Y., Okuyama, S., Sato, K., Takahashi, K., Sato, T., Kanno, I. ^{67}Ga tumor scanning and its mechanisms studied in rabbits. Radiology 100: 357-362, 1971.

26. Kramer, R.J., Goldstein, R.E., Hirshfeld, J.W., Johnston, G.S., Epstein, S.E. Visualization of acute myocardial infarction by the radionuclide gallium-67. Circulation 46 (No. 4, Suppl. No. 2): II - 20, 1972.

27. Lomas, F., Wagner, H.N. Accumulation of ionic ^{67}Ga in empyema of the gallbladder. Radiology 105: 689-692, 1972.

28. Gelrud, L.G., Arseneau, J.C., Johnston, G.S. Gallium-67 localization in experimental and clinical abscesses. Clin Res 20: 881, 1972.

29. Ito, Y., Okuyama, S., Awano, T., Takahashi, K., Sato, T., Kanno, I. Diagnostic evaluation of ^{67}Ga scanning of lung cancer and other diseases. Radiology 101: 355-362, 1971.

30. Anghileri, L.J. Studies on the accumulation mechanisms of radioisotopes used in tumor diagnosis. Strahlentherapie 142: 456-462, 1971.

31. Gunasekera, S.W., King, L.J., Lavender, P.J. The behavior of tracer gallium-67 towards serum proteins. Clin Chim Acta 39: 401-406, 1972.

32. Blair, D.C., Carroll, M., Carr, E.A., Fekety, F.R. ^{67}Ga-citrate for scanning experimental staphylococcal abscesses. J Nucl Med 14: 99-102, 1973.

33. Gelrud, L.G., Arseneau, J.C., Milder, M.S., Kramer, R.J., Swann, S.J., Canellos, G.P., Johnston, G.S. The kinetics of gallium-67 incorporation into inflammatory lesions: experimental and clinical studies. Submitted, J Lab Clin Med.

34. Small, R.C., Bennett, L.R. Normal ^{67}Ga scan. J Nucl Med 12: 394, 1971.

35. Larson, S.M., Schall, G.L. Gallium-67 concentration in human breast milk. JAMA 218: 257, 1971.

36. Lomas, F., Dibos, P.E., Wagner, H.N. Increased specificity of liver scanning with the use of ^{67}Ga citrate. N Engl J Med

286: 1323-1329, 1972.

37. Winchell, H.S., Sanchez, P.D., Watanabe, C.K., Hollander, L., Anger, H.O., McRae, J., Hayes, R.L., Edwards, C.L. Visualization of tumors in humans using ^{67}Ga-citrate and the Anger whole-body scanner, scintillation camera and tomographic scanner. J Nucl Med 11: 459-466, 1970.

38. Milder, M.S., Glick, J.H., Henderson, E.S., Johnston, G.S. ^{67}Ga scintigraphy in acute leukemia. Cancer. In press.

39. Peters, M.V. A study of survivals in Hodgkin's disease treated radiologically. Am J Roentgenol 63: 299-311, 1950.

40. Rosenberg, S.A. Report of the committee on the staging of Hodgkin's disease. Cancer Res 26: 1310, 1966.

41. Carbone, P.P., Kaplan, H.S., Musshoff, K., Smithers, D.W., Tubiana, M. Report of the committee on Hodgkin's disease staging classification. Cancer Res 31: 1860-1861, 1971.

42. Lee, Y.N., Say, C., Hori, J.M., Spratt, J.S. Clinical courses of Hodgkin's disease and other malignant lymphomas. Am J Roentgenol Radium Ther Nucl Med 117: 19-29, 1973.

43. Gough, J. Hodgkin's disease; a correlation of histopathology with survival. Int J Cancer 5: 273-281, 1970.

44. Kaplan, H.S. On the natural history, treatment, and prognosis of Hodgkin's disease. Harvey Lect Series 64: 215-259, 1968-1969.

45. DeVita, V.T., Canellos, G.P., Moxley, J.H. A decade of combination chemotherapy of advanced Hodgkin's disease. Cancer 30: 1495-1504, 1972.

46. Jones, S.E., Fuks, Z., Bull, M., Kadin, M.E., Dorfman, R.F., Kaplan, H.S., Rosenberg, S.A., Kim, H. Non-Hodgkin's lymphomas IV. Clinicopathologic correlation in 405 cases. Cancer 31: 806-823, 1973.

47. Rosenberg, S.A., Boiron, M., DeVita, V.T., Johnson, R.E., Lee, B.J., Ultmann, J.E., Viamonte, M. Report of the committee on Hodgkin's disease staging procedures. Cancer Res 31: 1862-1863, 1971.

48. Glatstein, E., Guernsey, J.M., Rosenberg, S.A., Kaplan, H.S. The value of laparotomy and splenectomy in the staging of Hodgkin's disease. Cancer 24: 709-718, 1969.

49. Milder, M.S., Larson, S.M., Bagley, C.M., DeVita, V.T., Johnson,
     R.E., Johnston, G.S. Liver-spleen scan in Hodgkin's disease.
     Cancer 31: 826-834, 1973.

50. Turner, D.A., Pinsky, S.M., Gottschalk, A., Hoffer, P.B.,
     Ultmann, J.E., Harper, P.V. The use of Ga-67 scanning in the
     staging of Hodgkin's disease. Radiology 104: 97-101, 1972.

51. Kay, D.N., McCready, V.R. Clinical isotope scanning using
     ^{67}Ga citrate in the management of Hodgkin's disease. Br J
     Radiol 45: 437-443, 1972.

52. Johnston, G.S., Teates, C.D., Benua, R.S., Edwards, C.L.,
     Kniseley, R.M. Gallium-67 citrate imaging in untreated
     Hodgkin's disease. J Nucl Med. In press.

53. Greenlaw, R.H., Weinstein, M.B., Brill, A.B., McBain, J.K.,
     Kniseley, R.M. Gallium-67 citrate imaging in untreated
     malignant lymphoma. J Nucl Med. In press.

54. Nash, A.G., Dance, D.R., McCready, V.R., Griffiths, J.D.
     Uptake of gallium-67 in colonic and rectal tumors. Br Med J
     3: 508-510, 1972.

55. Lavender, P.J., Lowe, J., Barker, J.R., Burn, J.I., Chaudhri,
     M.A. Gallium 67 citrate scanning in neoplastic and inflam-
     matory lesions. Br J Radiol 44: 361-366, 1971.

56. Suzuki, T., Honjo, I., Hamamoto, K., Kousaka, T., Torizuka, K.
     Positive scintiphotography of cancer of the liver with Ga^{67}
     citrate. Am J Roentgenol Radium Ther Nucl Med 113: 92-103,
     1971.

57. Lund, H.Z., Kraus, J.M. Melanotic tumors of the skin.
     Washington, D.C., Armed Forces Institute of Pathology, 1962
     (National Research Council, Committee of Pathology, Atlas of
     Pathology, Section 1, Fascicle 3).

58. Luce, J.K. Chemotherapy of malignant melanoma. Cancer 30:
     1604-1615, 1972.

59. Beierwaltes, W.H., Lieberman, L.M., Varma, V.M., Counsell, R.E.
     Visualizing human malignant melanoma and metastases. Use of
     chloroquine analog tagged with Iodine 125. JAMA 206: 97-
     102, 1968.

60. Hagler, W.S., Jarrett, W.H., Humphrey, W.T. The radioactive
     phosphorus uptake test in diagnosis of uveal melanoma. Arch
     Ophthalmol 83: 548-557, 1970.

61. Berelowitz, M., Blake, K.C.H. [67]Gallium in the detection and localization of tumours. S Afr Med J 45: 1351-1359, 1971.

62. Jones, A.E., Koslow, M., Johnston, G.S., Ommaya, A.K. 67-Ga citrate scintigraphy of brain tumors. Radiology 105: 693-697, 1972.

63. Henkin, R.E., Quinn, J.L., Weinberg, P.E. Adjunctive brain scanning with ^{67}Ga in metastases. Radiology 106: 595-599, 1973.

64. Kramer, R.J., Larson, S.M., Milder, M.S., Herdt, J.R., Johnson, R.E., DeVita, V.T., Johnston, G.S. Localization of [67]Gallium citrate in unsuspected sites of neoplastic disease. Proceedings of the International Atomic Energy Agency Symposium on Medical Radioisotope Scintigraphy. Monte Carlo, Principality of Monaco, October 23-28, 1972. In press.

65. Hartman, R.E., Hayes, R.L. The binding of gallium and indium by blood serum proteins. In 1967 Research Report, Medical Division, Oak Ridge Associated Universities, ORAU-106, Oak Ridge, p 120, 1967.

66. Mühe, E. Zur diagnostik des bronchialkarzinoms. Fortschr Roentgenstr Nuklearmed 115: 496-501, 1971.

67. Heller, H. Hirnszintigraphie mit [67-]gallium. Fortschr Roentgenstr Nuklearmed 117: 704-706, 1972.

68. Ramos, M., Jammers, W., Stahl, H.J. Szintigraphische tumordiagnostik mit 67 Ga-citrat. Fortschr Roentgenstr Nuklearmed 117: 689-697, 1972.

69. Edwards, C.L., Hayes, R.L., Nelson, B. The "normal" [67]Ga scan. J Nucl Med 13: 428-429, 1972.

70. Edwards, C.L., Hayes, R.L. Tumor scanning with ^{67}Ga citrate. Preliminary note. J Nucl Med 10: 103-105, 1969.

INDEX

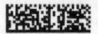